NATURAL BIRTH CONTROL
MADE SIMPLE

"The book is excellent. There is no other like it." — *Health Care Counselor, Family Planning Clinic, Decatur, Illinois*

"I am happy to finally see a book on NFP/FAM that is simple enough for a high school student to understand and yet comprehensive enough to adequately explain what is involved in the method. I also appreciate the authors' encouragement for people to attend a class by a certified instructor." — *R.N., Family Planning Clinic, Stockton, California*

"I love it! I have read every book on the subject and think it is unquestionably the best book on NFP ever written. I plan to use it for my classes at Planned Parenthood." — *Instructor, Planned Parenthood*

"This is an excellent resource. The best we've seen in quite some time." — *Health Educator, Health Department, Sumter, South Carolina*

"Enjoyed chapter on history. Book is simply written and very easily understood. Of all the books I've read, this is the first one that makes sense." — *R.N., Family Planning Clinic, Dover, New Hampshire*

"Your book is truly excellent. It is the best book on the subject." — *Professor, Women's Studies, Northeastern Illinois University*

"Fills a need and does it admirably. We are using it in our clinic as an extension of all birth control information. It is a must for all women." — *Counselor, Family Planning Clinic, Cincinnati, Ohio*

"I feel that the information was clearly and concisely explained. My clients have told me the book was easy to follow and the charts helpful to read." — *Fertility Awareness Instructor, Family Planning*

"Probably the best book on fertility awareness I've seen for the public." — *RNP, Family Planning Clinic, Laramie, Wyoming*

"Very excellent book on fertility. Wonderful educational drawings and text was clear and easily understandable, yet contained essential and interesting details. Thank you for this book." — *R.N., Center for Men, Arcata, California*

IMPORTANT NOTE

The material in this book is intended to provide an overview of fertility awareness and the use of natural family planning and fertility awareness methods for pregnancy prevention and achievement. Although this book has been prepared by experts in the field of fertility awareness, it does not purport to take the place of qualified medical advice and treatment when appropriate.

The author, editors, reviewers, and publishers cannot be held responsible for any error, omission, professional disagreement, outdated material, or adverse outcomes that derive from use of any of these treatments in a program of self-care or under the care of a licensed practitioner. Please contact your doctor and/or a fertility awareness instructor regarding medical matters and problems related to natural family planning and fertility awareness methods.

It is also important to note that, while this method of family planning is effective in preventing pregnancy, it provides absolutely no protection against sexually-transmitted diseases.

ORDERING

Trade bookstores in the U.S. and Canada please contact:

Publishers Group West
1700 Fourth Street, Berkeley CA 94710
Phone: (800) 788-3123   Fax: (510) 528-3444

Hunter House books are available at bulk discounts for textbook course adoptions; to qualifying community, health-care, and government organizations; and for special promotions and fund-raising. For details please contact:

Special Sales Department
Hunter House Inc., PO Box 2914, Alameda CA 94501-0914
Phone: (510) 865-5282   Fax: (510) 865-4295
E-mail: sales@hunterhouse.com

Individuals can order our books from most bookstores, by calling (800) 266-5592, or from our website at www.hunterhouse.com

Natural

Birth

Control

Made Simple

Barbara Kass-Annese, RN, CNP, MSN
and Hal C. Danzer, MD

Hunter House
PUBLISHERS

Hunter House Inc., Publishers
PO Box 2914
Alameda CA 94501-0914

LIBRARY OF CONGRESS CATALOGING-IN-PUBLICATION DATA

Kass-Annese, Barbara.
Natural birth control made simple / Barbara Kass-Annese and Hal C. Danzer.
p. cm.
Includes bibliographical references and index.
ISBN 0-89793-403-2 (pbk. : alk. paper) — ISBN 0-89793-404-0 (cloth : alk. paper)
1. Natural family planning—Popular works. I. Danzer, Hal. II. Title.

RG136.5 .K373 2003
613.9'434—dc21   2002151933

PROJECT CREDITS

Original illustrations by Tom Rachel, revised by Sparrow Fraenkel
Cover Design: Brian Dittmar Graphic Design
Book Production: Hunter House
Copy Editor: Ashley Chase
Proofreader: John David Marion
Indexer: Nancy D. Peterson
Acquisitions Editor: Jeanne Brondino
Editor: Alexandra Mummery
Publicity Coordinator: Earlita K. Chenault
Sales & Marketing Coordinator: Jo Anne Retzlaff
Customer Service Manager: Christina Sverdrup
Order Fulfillment: Lakdhon Lama
Administrator: Theresa Nelson
Computer Support: Peter Eichelberger
Publisher: Kiran S. Rana

Printed and Bound by Bang Printing, Brainerd, Minnesota

Manufactured in the United States of America

9   8   7   6   5   4   3   2   1   7th Edition   03   04   05   06   07

Contents

      Illnesses, Etc. 122
      Ovulation on Time 125
      Late or Delayed Ovulation 126
      No Ovulation 126
      The Basic Infertile Patterns of Cervical Mucus 128
      Special Circumstances Rules 134
      Causes of Anovulation 145
      Other Special Circumstances 154
      Some Final Tips on Special Circumstances and Mucus 156

11 The Fertility Awareness Method 158

12 The Advantages and Disadvantages of Natural Family
      Planning and Fertility Awareness Methods 164
      Should You Use Natural Family Planning? 164
      What Does Sexuality Mean? 166
      Do You Want a Pregnancy? 168
      How Does Natural Family Planning Fit into All of This? 170
      The Advantages of the Fertility Awareness Method 171
      A Few Last Words... 172

Sample NFP Contracts 173
      Sample Contract for the Woman 174
      Sample Contract for the Couple 175

      Bibliography 176

      Index 179

      Blank Fertility Awareness Chart 182

List of Illustrations

Acknowledgments

The authors express their thanks to:

John Altamura
Bart Andrews
Joe Bectol
Dana Chalberg
Blake Conway
Gareth Esersky
Michelle Martino
H. Roy Matlen
F. Clyde Petersen
Kiran Rana
Sherri Robb
Barbara S. Rollins

who made *Natural Birth Control Made Simple* and its predecessors, *The Fertility Awareness Handbook*, *The Fertility Awareness Workbook*, and *Patterns*, possible.

Introduction

Natural Birth Control Made Simple was written for several reasons:

- ✤ to offer you the most accurate and up-to-date information about reproduction and fertility;
- ✤ to give you easy, step-by-step instructions on how to use natural, safe, and very effective choices for pregnancy prevention; and
- ✤ to give you extremely vital information that will help you conceive if you trying to become pregnant now or planning a pregnancy in the future.

It was also written to help you learn what is normal for you. If you use the information for this reason and no other, you are helping yourself in a very special way because you will be better prepared to meet your own health-care needs.

This book is entitled *Natural Birth Control Made Simple* for a very important reason: It is written to "get the word out" that there are ways to prevent pregnancy **naturally** and **simply**! Natural birth control, also commonly known nowadays as Natural Family Planning (NFP), is based on the natural changes in fertility that take place in a woman every month. These changes can be tracked using indicators called fertility signs, so that a woman can determine the days during each menstrual cycle when she is fertile and can become pregnant or is infertile and cannot become pregnant. When a couple wants to use NFP methods for pregnancy prevention, they choose to abstain from intercourse on the woman's fertile days.

NFP methods have been around for quite some time and unfortunately have gained somewhat of a reputation for being difficult to understand and use. It's time to change all that! You will find that *Natural*

Birth Control Made Simple is written and designed to provide you with NFP information in a clear and easy-to-use format so you can understand it fully and use it in many rewarding ways throughout your life. The book also provides specific instruction in the use of another family planning option known as the Fertility Awareness Method (FAM). Based on the same fertility cycle information as NFP, FAM gives a couple the option of having intercourse using a barrier and/or spermicidal contraceptive method on the days the woman *can* become pregnant.

Natural Birth Control Made Simple has a clear logic to it. It begins with a brief introduction to and history of natural family planning, followed by chapters on how the reproductive systems of women and men work. All of this basic knowledge is meant to help you increase your awareness of the normal and natural changes of the reproductive cycle.

Following the chapters on basics, there is a detailed explanation and description of the body's fertility signs. Knowing exactly what fertility signs are and how they work, as well as why they work, will give you confidence with your own personal method of family planning.

Because some couples will use fertility signs to help them become pregnant, the subject of infertility and instructions on how to use fertility signs to increase the possibility of pregnancy are discussed next. Since there are only a few days each menstrual or fertility cycle in which pregnancy is possible, it is crucial to have intercourse during these days. When I worked in an infertility practice, I was upset to learn of the number of women who weren't becoming pregnant **only** because they were not having intercourse during the right time! It is for this reason that a chapter is dedicated to teaching the way in which NFP is used to help women become pregnant. It does not, however, include in-depth information about infertility for a very real reason. The field of infertility is complex and ever changing. If you find at some point that you are in need of information about various aspects of infertility, please obtain the best resources possible, ones written by fertility specialists.

It can't be emphasized enough how important it is to obtain information from health-care professionals who "live and breathe" the world of infertility—fertility specialists. By doing this, you can obtain the best and most accurate information possible. Many books have been written by fertility experts, and organizations exist that are dedicated to helping women and couples who are having difficulty conceiving. The names of a few of these infertility resources have been included in the Bibliography at the end of this book.

As you begin reading about the facts of fertility awareness and end with a consideration of your own feelings, we hope you find this awareness and information rewarding and enriching. It's now time to begin your own personal fertility journey. Enjoy!

1

Natural Family Planning and Fertility Awareness Methods: What Are They?

What is your family planning goal right now? Is it to delay having a child for a while? Is it to prevent pregnancy for the rest of your childbearing years because you do not want any children or any more children?

Is it to become pregnant now or at some point in the future?

If you want to prevent pregnancy, how do you want to do this? Perhaps you are comfortable using an abstinence-based method of family planning, meaning you won't have intercourse during the days you can become pregnant. Or, perhaps you use or are planning to use condoms or some other barrier and/or spermicidal method of contraception and want to use them only when they are needed, meaning only during your fertile days.

Regardless of your answer to these questions, you have something in common with all women who decide to learn about their fertility in ways that will help them reach their family planning goal. All of you must begin by learning the same information. This information is called fertility awareness education.

Fertility awareness (FA) education includes the most current and accurate information about reproduction and fertility signs, the naturally occurring changes in your body you experience from one menstrual period to the next. Fertility signs change in predictable and dependable ways for most healthy women in their reproductive years. Because of this, they can be used to accurately identify the days a woman can and cannot become pregnant:

Days you can become pregnant = Fertile days

Days you cannot become pregnant = Infertile days

If you want to prevent pregnancy by choosing to abstain from intercourse during the fertile days, you will be using what is known as natural family planning (NFP).

NFP is actually a name that was chosen over thirty years ago by people involved in the research and teaching of abstinence-based methods. Natural family planning seemed an appropriate name for methods that combine the use of monitoring fertility signs and abstinence from intercourse during fertile days, because they are based on using changes in **naturally occurring** signs and symptoms of fertility to identify fertile and infertile days. There are several NFP methods available for use, and you will learn about all of them in later chapters.

Approximately twenty years ago, several of us working in the field of family planning discussed the idea that, while fertile and infertile days could be accurately determined by observing fertility signs, a woman or couple should have other choices during the fertile days besides abstinence. Abstinence might not fit into some people's lifestyles. These people should be able to use a different birth control method, such as condoms, diaphragms, or spermicide, during the fertile days. We decided to use the term *fertility awareness method* (FAM) when such contraceptive methods are used during the fertile days instead of abstinence.

Regardless of whether NFP or FAM is used, the significant point is this: Your body reveals fertility signs that enable you to identify the fertile and infertile days during each menstrual or fertility cycle. This is a natural language that is spoken by your body. *By learning this language, you can join the thousands of women and men who are now enjoying these alternative approaches to family planning!*

2

The Evolution of Natural Family Planning and Fertility Awareness Methods

Since the beginning of recorded history, people have sought reliable methods to prevent pregnancy and enhance fertility. Women beyond the healthy childbearing years or women who were ill were not expected to bear children. The woman who experienced repeated stillbirths or very difficult deliveries often sought to avoid future pregnancies. Times of war, famine, or inability to adequately provide for the health and safety of a child were also important factors in the choice to delay pregnancy. As you can see from these examples, people throughout the ages had many of the same reasons for pregnancy prevention as we do today.

How Have People Attempted to Prevent Pregnancy?

Beginning with pre-Biblical times, people have used abstinence, breastfeeding, withdrawal, magical potions, charms, and herbal mixtures to prevent pregnancy.

During the time of the ancient Hebrews, one method used was a spongy substance placed inside the vagina to block sperm. Greek and Roman literature tells us of many methods of birth control, such as the use of vaginal suppositories made from honey and peppermint juice.

During the Middle Ages, both European and Islamic cultures used a number of recipes, many magical, to avoid pregnancy. One unusual recipe instructed a woman who did not want to become pregnant to soak a piece of cloth in the oil of a barberry tree and place it on the left side of her forehead. Other supposed methods of birth control included eating beans on an empty stomach; rubbing tar on the penis prior to intercourse; douching with solutions made of lemon juice; placing algae, seaweed, or the husks of mahogany nuts inside the vagina before intercourse; carrying a child's tooth; and drinking thyme and lavender tea.

Since fertility was usually not understood, it was often considered mystical. Slowly, as a truer understanding about the facts of physiology and reproduction emerged, science and technology began to take the place of magical interpretations.

Around the middle of the eighteenth century, although potions and ceremonies continued to be used, modern mechanical forms of birth control began emerging. The condom was one of the first of these to be introduced.

The birth control movement in America had begun by 1828. Techniques included withdrawal, using a vaginal sponge made from sheep's wool or silk, and using douching solutions made from white oak bark, green tea, or vinegar and water. Although the use of the diaphragm emerged in Holland during the early 1880s, it was not introduced to American women until the early 1920s. Between the 1920s and 1930s the rhythm method, Gräfenberg intrauterine silver ring, and spermicides began to be used. From that point on, several types of intrauterine devices were developed. Finally "the Pill" entered the mainstream of American life during the 1960s, and several hormonal methods have been developed since then. Today, hormones are administered in the form of pills, injectables, patches, and rings to prevent pregnancy.

What Is the History of Natural Family Planning?

We know from the past to the present, in various areas throughout the world, women have used and continue to use breastfeeding as a natural means of child spacing. Yet compared to the thousands of real and "magical" methods of contraception that have evolved and been recorded, little has been written about other forms of natural family planning. Some groups of Africans, Native Americans, and others appear to have had some knowledge of their fertility cycles and practiced abstinence from intercourse, but there is little information available on their traditional birth control practices. What we do know is that some women in traditional cultures did use one of the major fertility signs, cervical mucus, as a means to achieve or avoid pregnancy, and it is still used by them today.

Over 150 years ago a researcher, Dr. Theodore Bischoff, found eggs present in the uterus and fallopian tubes of a female dog while the dog was bleeding, or "in heat." Because of this discovery he assumed that women must also have eggs present during their menstrual bleeding. Therefore, he believed that women became pregnant if they had intercourse during their periods. As a result of his findings, a natural birth control schedule was developed. It stated that if pregnancy was to be avoided, intercourse should not occur during the menstrual period, as well as 5 days before it and 9 days after it. It was considered that these were the days when the woman could become pregnant. We now know that just the opposite is true!

This "natural birth control" continued to be practiced until the 1930s, and countless women became pregnant trying to use this totally incorrect information.

However, not all past information on fertility signs was incorrect. As early as 1857, there were descriptions of women who believed they could tell when they were ovulating because once a month they experienced internal aching or a painful feeling in the area of the ovaries. (Ovulation is the release of the egg from the ovary.)

This pain with ovulation continued to be discussed and written about for years. In 1935, Dr. Cyrus Anderson wrote a paper entitled, "Teaching the Patient to Observe Symptoms of Ovulation." In it he discussed ovulation pain and how women could be taught to recognize it.

Ovulation pain, as you will soon learn, can be used by some women as a fertility sign. One of the other fertility signs you will learn about is the temperature of the body at rest, known as basal body temperature. It was studied as early as 1876 by Dr. Marie Putnam Jacobi. She found that the basal body temperature increases and decreases at certain times during the menstrual or fertility cycle and these temperature changes follow a very distinct pattern.

Researchers in the 1800s also wrote about another fertility sign—cervical mucus, the substance made in the cervix (the bottom part of the uterus). In fact, around the mid-1800s it was observed that this mucus changed in amount and quality throughout the menstrual or fertility cycle. These observations led researchers to believe that a particular kind of mucus was needed to achieve a pregnancy. This belief, of course, later proved to be scientific fact!

Finally, in 1929, the rhythm method was developed when two men on opposite sides of the world, and working independently of each other, discovered that an egg is released from the ovary approximately fourteen days before each menstrual period.. This discovery formed the basis of the Ogina-Knaus Calendar Rhythm Method, named after the two discoverers, Dr. Kyusaku Ogina and Dr. Hermann Knaus. The rhythm method has been shown to be very effective for the woman who experiences consistently regular cycles. However, unlike modern natural family planning methods, it does not take into account that a woman's fertile days can begin earlier or later than usual. This has contributed to unplanned pregnancies for some rhythm method users. In addition, the rhythm method usually requires longer periods of abstinence from intercourse than the modern methods of natural family planning.

In 1962, Dr. William Hartman found that sperm could live in the woman's body for three days, while the egg survives for one day after being released from the ovary. This added up to a four-day period of time during the menstrual or fertility cycle when a woman could become pregnant. We now know that if the proper conditions are present in the woman's body, sperm may live and remain capable of fertilizing the egg for a period of up to five days. This means that there are approximately six to seven days during the menstrual or fertility cycle when a pregnancy is possible.

During the 1960s, an Australian team of physicians, Drs. John and Evelyn Billings, sought to develop a method of natural family planning that would be more accurate than the rhythm method. They conducted extensive research on cervical mucus, which led to the development of the Billings Method, also known as the cervical mucus method or the ovulation method. This method is based on using observations of one fertility sign, the cervical mucus, to determine the fertile and infertile days of the menstrual or fertility cycle.

Another method of natural family planning was also being used around the time the Billings Method was introduced. It was called the sympto-thermal method because it includes the use of several symptoms of ovulation and basal body temperature to determine the infertile and fertile days of the menstrual or fertility cycle.

All this adds up to the fact that reliable methods of natural family planning, the ovulation and sympto-thermal methods, have been used by people throughout the world for over thirty-five years!

How Effective Are These Methods of Natural Family Planning?

Before answering this question, it is important to acknowledge that a couple's feelings about pregnancy play a very important role in how a method of birth control is used. Women and men who are motivated to prevent a pregnancy tend to use a method more carefully, and careful use means fewer pregnancies.

Because of this fact and others, effectiveness rates, or how successful a method of birth control is, are discussed in two ways. One is the *perfect* or *theoretical* effectiveness rate. This type of effectiveness rate tells us how well a method works when used perfectly. In other words, no mistakes are made on the parts of the clinician or instructor providing the birth control method or the person using the method. The second type of effectiveness rate is called *actual* or *use* effectiveness rate. This is the real-life effectiveness of the method, taking into account human error made by the user of the method, the clinician, or the instructor.

For example, if a couple using NFP chose to have intercourse during a fertile time and the woman became pregnant, this would be called a user pregnancy. A pregnancy may also occur because of the inability of the couple to understand the method, and this may be due to the teacher, the couple, or a combination of both. These unplanned pregnancies would be counted toward the method's actual or use effectiveness rate.

If a couple using NFP perfectly becomes pregnant, this is a theoretical or perfect use pregnancy—a failure of the method itself to prevent pregnancy. Every method that exists today has a perfect user pregnancy rate. For whatever reason, even when the pill is taken every day or when a vasectomy seems to be performed perfectly, some women will eventually become pregnant!

A three-year study, supported by the Department of Health, Education, and Welfare, and completed in 1979 at Cedar-Sinai Medical Center in Los Angeles, compared the effectiveness of the ovulation method with that of the sympto-thermal method. Over 1,200 couples participated in this study. It was found that the ovulation method had a user effectiveness rate of approximately 78 percent. This means that 22 out of every 100 women who began use of the method, and who did not stop using it for any reason, became pregnant within one year. The sympto-thermal method was determined to be approximately 89 percent use effective, which means that out of every 100 women who began use of this method and did not stop using it for any reason, 11 became pregnant within one year. The results of this particular study are generally similar to many others that have been conducted throughout the world.

Most of the pregnancies in this study occurred because people took chances and had intercourse during the fertile time, did not understand the use of the methods, or did not follow other instructions necessary for the effective use of these two methods.

The reason why the couples using the sympto-thermal (S-T) method experienced a lower number of pregnancies is not completely understood. However, the Cedar-Sinai study and others, in addition to our own experience in working with these methods, suggest that for many people the S-T method is easier to teach, to learn, and to use properly. The findings of this particular study, in addition to many others, have consistently suggested that the perfect use effectiveness rates of both methods are approximately equal. When instructed correctly by the teachers, in combination with the couples' understanding and proper use of the methods, the effectiveness rates are approximately 98 percent.

Other studies conducted since that time have shown comparable rates. The effectiveness rates of the natural family planning methods are comparable with almost all of the other methods of contraception.

Effectiveness of Several Contraceptive Methods

	Theoretical Effectiveness	Use Effectiveness
Hormonal Methods	99+%	90–94%
Condom and Spermicide	99+%	95%
Intrauterine Device	97–99%	95%
Condom	97%	90%
Diaphragm	97%	83%
Spermicides	97%	78%

Only a couple of very small FAM studies have been conducted, none of which have completely documented the effectiveness of the use of barrier and spermicidal methods of contraception during the fertile time. Many family planning professionals believe, however, that the effectiveness rate of using a barrier and/or spermicidal method only during the fertile days should be about the same as the rates achieved when the diaphragm, condom, and spermicide are used in traditional fashion (i.e., used every time intercourse takes place throughout the menstrual or fertility cycle).

Many health-care professionals believe that because FAM includes the use of these other methods only during the fertile time, people may actually use them more conscientiously and correctly, resulting in fewer unplanned pregnancies.

The reasons people choose to use natural family planning or fertility awareness methods are certainly varied and complex. To some, NFP is a way of life. It is not only a method of birth control, but a total way that a woman and man relate to each other, spiritually, emotionally, and physically. NFP is also a method that is compatible with the teachings of certain religions. For others, NFP is used because it is in keeping with their beliefs about their health. Some people desire to eliminate as many chemicals as possible from their lifestyle. And for some, natural family planning is the only method of birth control they can or want to use, due to problems with other methods of birth control. The numbers of people using the fertility awareness method appear to be growing because it seems that they wish to use the natural language of the body in combination with a method of birth control they are comfortable with. In the end, the method chosen will depend upon a number of factors, including the physical, emotional, sexual, and spiritual needs and beliefs of the person/couple.

Now that we've briefly introduced natural family planning and fertility awareness methods to you, and given you an idea of how poorly reproduction was understood in the past, it's time to begin learning how much better reproduction is understood today.

3

The Man and His Fertility

A man's fertility is constant. This means that millions of sperm are always ready and waiting to fulfill their only purpose—to meet with an egg. Well into his seventies or even older, a man has the ability to father a child any day or night, at any time of the day or night! The man's constant fertility is, to a great degree, made possible through ongoing communication between parts of the brain and the **testes**. The testes are the sex glands of the man and the major source of the male hormone **testosterone**. They are also the place where sperm are made and begin to mature. They then travel to the **epididymus** where they complete their maturation process.

In general, **hormones** play a major role in controlling how the body works. We wouldn't exist without them. There are many different hormones produced by various glands in the body, such as the thyroid and adrenal glands. Hormones are considered powerful chemical messengers: Once they are produced by a particular gland, they travel through the bloodstream to the parts of the body they are supposed to reach. Hormones help these parts work in specific ways. When it comes to a man's fertility, just the right amount of hormones must be made to ensure that enough healthy sperm are produced and mature on a continuous basis. Though the testes are the major source of testosterone needed for this task, they cannot work unless they receive messages from hormones produced by the pituitary gland.

The **pituitary gland** is located at the base of the brain and is responsible for continuously sending hormonal messages to the testes so that they are able to work properly. This gland becomes more active

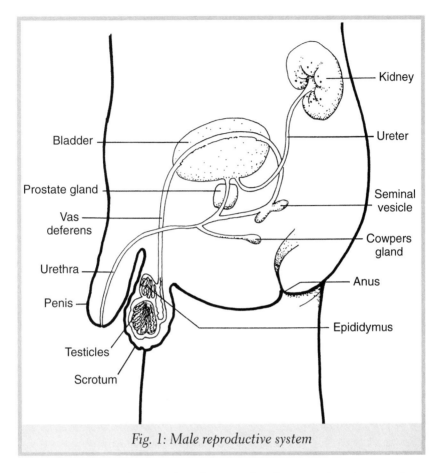

Fig. 1: Male reproductive system

around the time a boy reaches the age of eight to twelve. As a result, a time of physical and emotional change known as **puberty** begins, and it lasts about four years. During these years, testosterone plays an important part in the development of the boy's body. For example, testosterone causes the growth of body hair and sex organs, including the penis. Sexual feelings also begin to increase under the influence of testosterone. This is the time a boy begins to experience nocturnal emissions, known as "wet dreams"—a normal involuntary ejaculation that occurs when the boy is asleep. (Ejaculation is the release of semen from the penis.)

During puberty, the pituitary gland sends a message to the testes. As a result of this message, the testes begin to produce sperm and testosterone. The testes are a pair of oval shaped organs that produce at least 50,000,000 sperm each day. They are protected by two sacs of loose, thin tissue known as the **scrotum**. The scrotum and testes are located on the outside of the man's body for a very specific reason—to keep them cooler than normal body temperature. Sperm can only be produced at this cooler temperature. Once sperm are produced in the testes, they travel to the **epididymis**. This is the area where sperm become fully developed and wait until they begin their journey through the rest of the man's reproductive system.

When ejaculation is about to occur, sperm leave the epididymis and move along the **vas deferens**, a pair of 20-inch-long tubes that carry them past the **seminal vesicles**. These sac-like structures produce seminal fluid that mixes with the sperm. The mixture of sperm and seminal fluid continues traveling through the vas deferens, which goes around the side of the bladder, to the **prostate gland**. This gland is the size and shape of an acorn and produces a thin, milky fluid that nourishes the sperm. When sperm mixes with fluid from the seminal vesicles and prostate gland, semen is formed. The semen moves into the passageway of the **ejaculatory duct** and then travels through the urethra and out of the man's body. The urethra is the tube that runs through the center of the penis. Usually the urethra serves as the exit for urine from the man's body, but during ejaculation urine cannot come out of the bladder. Instead, only semen is able to travel through the urethra.

The **Cowpers glands** are glands located within the man's reproductive system and are important to discuss because they produce a few drops of fluid shortly before ejaculation. This fluid travels through the urethra. It can't be felt by the man, but the small amount of fluid can be seen at the tip of the man's penis shortly before he ejaculates. Since the urethra is usually a passageway for urine, its environment is usually acidic. Sperm cannot survive in an acidic environment. Fluid from the Cowpers glands flows through the urethra in order to change its acid environment to one in which sperm can live. For years, health-care professionals were taught that the Cowpers glands fluid contained millions of healthy sperm. It was therefore believed that if the tip of a man's penis with the fluid on it came into contact with a woman's vaginal area during her fertile days, sperm could swim up inside her reproductive system and meet with an egg. Fortunately, today we know that Cowpers glands fluid cannot cause pregnancy. It is important to note, however, that a woman *can* become pregnant without having intercourse. If a man ejaculates semen at or near a woman's vaginal opening during her fertile days, pregnancy can result. The entire process of ejaculation is complex and controlled by messages being sent between the man's spinal cord, brain, and reproductive system. Blood must fill up the tissues of the penis so that it can become firm. This happens as a result of sexual arousal. When a man has reached a high level of sexual arousal, contractions begin in the muscles and other parts of the reproductive system. The contractions cause the sperm to leave the epididymus, travel through and past the parts mentioned above, and push the semen out through the urethra.

What is the most important fact to remember about a man's fertility?
The man is fertile every day from puberty through age 70 or longer!

4

The Woman and Her Fertility

The woman's fertility pattern is quite different from the man's. While the man is fertile every day, the woman is fertile approximately five to seven days during each menstrual or fertility cycle. To understand why this is so is to learn how the woman's reproductive system works. This can be done by first looking at the part of the system located on the outside of the woman's body. This part is called the external genitalia, or outer reproductive organs (see Figure 2 on page 19).

External Female Reproductive Anatomy

The **mons veneris** (named after Venus, the goddess of love)is a pad of fatty tissue that covers the pubic bone and at puberty becomes covered with pubic hair. It helps to protect the internal reproductive organs. Below it is the **vaginal opening**, or the entrance to the **vaginal canal**. This opening allows for the final exit of menstrual blood from the body. The vaginal canal widens to allow for intercourse and also expands during the birth of a baby. Usually, a baby girl is born with a paper-thin tissue that covers the vaginal opening yet has a small opening in it. This allows for the normal vaginal discharge and menstrual blood to flow out of the vagina. The tissue, known as the **hymen,** can easily be stretched and torn by insertion of a tampon, finger, or penis. Once this occurs, irregular-looking pieces of the hymen are left around the vaginal opening. These pieces are known as the **hymenal tags.**

Located on either side of the vaginal opening are two sets of vaginal lips. The outer set is made of fatty tissue covered with skin that contains oil-producing glands. These outer lips are covered, to some degree, with

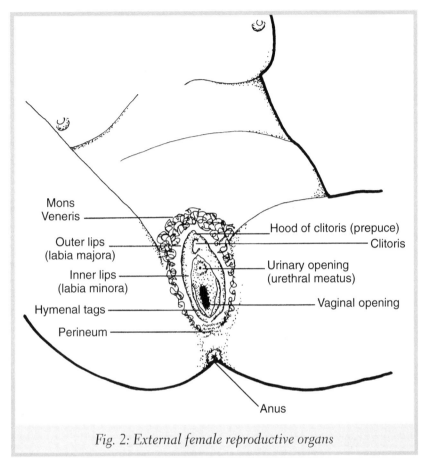

Mons Veneris

Outer lips (labia majora)

Inner lips (labia minora)

Hymenal tags

Perineum

Hood of clitoris (prepuce)

Clitoris

Urinary opening (urethral meatus)

Vaginal opening

Anus

Fig. 2: External female reproductive organs

pubic hair. The inner set of lips are hairless and do not contain oil-producing glands. This set is made of folds of soft skin. Together, the **labia majora** (outer lips) and **labia minora** (inner lips) protect the vaginal opening when a woman is not sexually aroused. When a woman does become sexually aroused, blood flows into the vaginal lips, causing them to fill with blood and flatten out away from the vagina—allowing for sexual activity. The **clitoris,** a small organ located below the mons veneris and above the vaginal opening, is made of the same kind of tissue as the penis. As with the penis, the clitoris becomes filled with blood during sexual arousal, causing it to become firm and erect. It contains many nerve endings which make it the main area of sexual arousal for many women. The clitoris is protected by a covering called the clitoral **hood,** which is formed by the joining of the inner lips above the clitoris.

Below the clitoris and above the vaginal entrance is the urinary opening, or **urethral meatus.** This opening is the entrance to the urethra, a tube leading to the bladder. The urinary opening serves as the passageway for the urine to travel from the bladder to the outside of the body. Below the vaginal opening is the **perineum.** This area of tissue is often cut during the birth of a baby to allow the baby easier passage out of the vaginal opening. The perineum separates the vaginal opening from the **anus,** the muscular opening of the **rectum** that serves as the exit for the body's solid waste materials.

The **vulva** is the name given to all of the outer parts or external genitalia that we've just described. Women often wonder if their vulva looks normal. The amount of pubic hair, size of the vaginal lips, and shape and size of the clitoris are unique to each woman. If a woman places a mirror between her thighs, she can see these parts. The woman comfortable doing this can become better acquainted with her body. She can learn what is normal for her. In other words, a woman who takes the time to look and touch these various parts of her body can learn to feel comfortable with her own body and gain a fuller understanding, awareness, and appreciation of it. This may help her overcome any uncomfortable feelings she may have about the outside of her reproductive system. It can also be an important health-care practice. In fact, it is now recommended that women regularly examine their vulvar area once a month just as they regularly examine their breasts. If anything unusual is seen or felt, it should be evaluated by a clinician.

Internal Female Reproductive Organs

As we have mentioned, many of the external parts of the woman's reproductive system help to protect the internal reproductive organs (Figure 3, page 21). The internal reproductive organs work together to enable a woman to become pregnant and nourish the pregnancy through nine months of development.

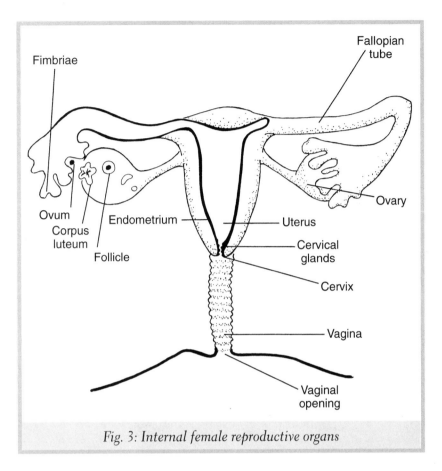

Fig. 3: Internal female reproductive organs

The **uterus** is a hollow, muscular organ that is somewhat pear-shaped. A woman's uterus is only about 3 inches long when she is not pregnant. There is a small space inside the uterus called the **endometrial cavity.** The innermost lining of the cavity is called the **endometrium.** During each normal menstrual or fertility cycle, this lining becomes rich in the blood supply and nutrients necessary for the growth of a healthy pregnancy.

The bottom part of the uterus is the **cervix,** which is located at the back of the vagina. Part of the cervix usually looks like a very small ball with an opening in the middle of it. For a woman who has never delivered a baby vaginally, the opening is very small, only about the size of the tip of a pen or pencil. For a woman who has had a vaginal delivery, the way the opening looks will depend on how the cervical opening was changed by the delivery process. For example, sometimes as the baby passes through the cervix during delivery, the cervix is stretched and can be torn to some degree. This can cause the opening to look like the mouth of a fish. Sometimes the cervix looks as though it has been divided into two or more parts. The next time you have a gynecological exam, if you are interested in knowing the shape of your cervix and opening, you could ask your health-care provider to either show you your cervix by using a mirror or draw you a picture of your cervix.

A 4–6-inch elastic, muscular tube is the connection between the cervix and the vaginal opening. Commonly called the **vaginal canal** or **birth canal**, this tube has the ability to expand during sexual arousal, allowing sexual intercourse. When a woman is sexually aroused, the amount of blood in the blood vessels in the tissues of the vagina increases. This causes the production of a slippery liquid, which lubricates the vaginal canal so that intercourse is comfortable. If a woman has an orgasm, vaginal and uterine muscles contract, as do muscles around the reproductive organs. (Please see the Bibliography for resources if you would like detailed information about the changes in men's and women's bodies during lovemaking and orgasm.)

One ovary is attached to each side of the uterus. The **ovaries** are the woman's sex glands and each is about the size and shape of an almond. Just as a man's testes produce hormones and sperm, a woman's ovaries produce hormones and are the place where eggs are formed and mature. The eggs cells are formed before the woman herself is born! In fact, when the female fetus has developed for about five months, 7 million immature egg cells are found in its ovaries. It is at this point that all the eggs cells a woman will ever have are present. After birth, her ovaries will not make any more of these.

The fascinating thing about egg cells is that from five months into fetal development until menopause, anywhere from 100 to 1,000 will be growing at any one time. A group will grow for a short period of time, then stop growing. Once each group of egg cells stops growing, these eggs will never be able to grow again, and they "die." This means that the number of eggs in a woman's body is always decreasing. As we have noted, a female fetus of five months has 7 million immature egg cells in its ovaries. In the four months between that time and birth, the number of egg cells has fallen from 7 million to only 2 million! By the time a girl reaches puberty, the number of egg cells in her ovaries has been reduced to about 400,000. By the time the mid-thirties are reached, the number has been reduced even further to about 100,000. Around the age of fifty-one, when menstruation stops for the average woman, the number of egg cells is very low. Perhaps only a couple of hundred are left, and they no longer mature and leave the ovary. When ovulation stops and a woman has no longer menstruated for one year, she has reached menopause and her reproductive years have ended.

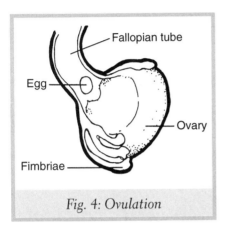

Fig. 4: Ovulation

Another interesting fact about the process of eggs cells growing and "dying" throughout a woman's lifetime is that it rarely stops. Even when a woman is pregnant or using hormonal methods of contraception, this is still taking place.

If egg cells are continuously growing and dying, how can a woman ever become pregnant? Pregnancy is only possible when one of the egg cells in the group that are growing is chosen to continue to develop into a mature egg and leave the ovary. The process of the egg leaving the ovary is called **ovulation**.

About two weeks before a woman menstruates, usually one egg leaves the ovary and is picked up by one of the **fallopian tubes**. The fallopian tubes are a pair of narrow, muscular passageways. They are thin and about 4 inches in length, and they have finger-like ends called **fimbriae**. The fimbriae encircle the ovary and pick up the egg. The egg will travel to the outer portion of the tube, where it will wait for about 24 hours. The egg cannot be fertilized unless sperm are waiting for it in the outer portion of the fallopian tube, or sperm make it to the egg within a 24-hour time period. After 24 hours, an unfertilized egg will be absorbed in the fallopian tube. It does not leave the uterus with menstrual blood. However, if the egg is fertilized, it will begin a journey of approximately one week down the fallopian tube into the uterus, where it will attach itself and continue to develop. The attachment of the egg to the lining of the uterus is called **implantation** (Figure 5, below).

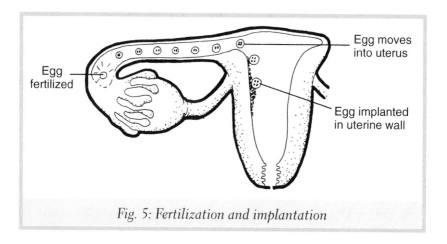

Fig. 5: Fertilization and implantation

If a woman doesn't become pregnant, the lining changes to allow the blood that has been building up for a possible pregnancy to leave the uterus. When this happens, the blood flows out through the cervix, travels down the vaginal canal, and exits through the vaginal opening.

As we mentioned above, the cervical opening is usually the size of the tip of a pen in a woman who has not had a vaginal delivery. However, the cervical opening widens at various times for different reasons. For instance, during menstruation this opening will widen to about the size of the tip of your pinky finger so that the blood can easily flow out of the uterus. This widening during menstruation occurs to some degree even when the cervix has already been widened to some degree by a vaginal delivery. The cervical opening also widens during ovulation, close to the time the egg is to come out of the ovary. This allows the sperm to travel easily into the cervix so that it can continue on its journey to the outer part of the fallopian tube and meet with an egg. The cervical opening also widens considerably during the vaginal birth of a baby. And finally, the cervical opening widens shortly after orgasm to be about as wide as it is during menstruation and ovulation. Some believe this helps a woman become pregnant. However, research hasn't shown this to be the case, particularly because a large number of women don't have orgasm during intercourse and still become pregnant without any difficulty.

Puberty and the Fertility Cycle

Ovulation begins at some point during **puberty**, the process by which a girl reaches physical and sexual maturity. For most young girls puberty begins between the ages of eight and thirteen. As with the boy, the process lasts about four years. Generally, the first sign of puberty is breast development, followed by growth of underarm and pubic hair. One of the last events of puberty is the start of menstrual bleeding. Although the beginning of menstrual bleeding means the ovaries have reached an adult level of development, some girls don't ovulate regularly or at all for one to two years after this first menstrual period. Once the eggs begin to be released, the young girl is fertile and can become pregnant.

The series of changes a woman's body constantly goes through, from the first day menstrual bleeding begins to the day before it begins again is commonly known as the **menstrual cycle**. Usually one egg leaves the ovary during each menstrual cycle. By the time a woman reaches menopause, about 400 will have been released.

A menstrual or fertility cycle always begins the first day any sign of menstrual bleeding appears, even if it is only spotting or a light flow of blood, and ends the day before menstrual bleeding begins again. For example, let's say Mary's menstrual bleeding began April 1. Her next menstrual bleeding began April 30. Therefore, her menstrual or fertility cycle during April was 29 days long.

Menstrual bleeding is the most visible part of the menstrual cycle. Most women are brought up to believe menstrual bleeding is the "main event," or the most important part of the cycle. The cycle is even named after menstruation. Yet, when you think about it, menstrual bleeding is only the beginning of a new cycle and means a woman did not become pregnant. The real purpose of the cycle is to prepare the woman's body for pregnancy and to allow ovulation to take place. *Ovulation, or the release of the egg from the ovary, is the MAIN EVENT of the menstrual cycle.* This cycle is a time in which a woman's body prepares for fertility! Because of this, we believe using the name **fertility cycle** in the place of "menstrual cycle" is more accurate and appropriate, particularly in the context of learning NFP.

The fertility cycle spans many days. Although a cycle can be somewhat shorter or longer, it usually ranges from 24–35 days in length. It is not unusual for a woman's fertility cycles to vary in length about 2–7 days from cycle to cycle. For example, the same woman may have cycles that are 25 days long, other cycles 27 days long, and still other cycles 32 days long. And that is okay—it is normal for her. It is also normal for the number of days on which menstrual bleeding occurs as well as the amount of bleeding to change with different cycles.

Events of the Fertility Cycle

A combination of events takes place throughout the fertility cycle that enables a woman to become pregnant. About the time menstrual bleeding begins, a part of the brain and the **pituitary gland,** a gland at the base of the brain, begin to communicate with each other and the ovaries so that several eggs can begin to grow. This communication is made possible by hormones produced by the pituitary gland and ovaries. The hormones travel through the bloodstream sending messages that enable eggs to grow as they should and enable the woman's reproductive system to prepare for the possibility of pregnancy.

Communication between the pituitary gland and ovaries causes the following:

1. The ovaries receive a message to start growing several of their immature egg cells.

2. As the egg cells are maturing, other cells that surround them are beginning to make hormones, including **estrogen**, the major female hormone. The egg cells combined with the cells that surround them are called a **follicle**.

3. As each egg cell matures in its follicle, cells in the follicle make more and more estrogen.

4. At some point, usually one egg will be chosen to grow to maturity and come out of the ovary (no one knows how this happens). The rest of the eggs stop growing.

5. Estrogen causes the lining of the uterus to grow and develop the proper blood supply and nutrients necessary for the fertilized egg to attach to the lining of the uterus.

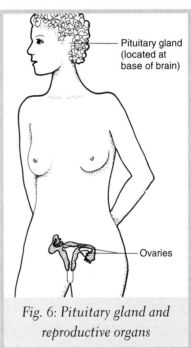

Pituitary gland (located at base of brain)

Ovaries

Fig. 6: Pituitary gland and reproductive organs

6. As the lining of the uterus is preparing for the possibility of pregnancy, estrogen causes the cells in the cervix to begin to make cervical mucus. As the time of ovulation nears, this mucus becomes very **fertile cervical mucus.** Fertile mucus contains a good amount of water and several substances that sperm love! When in this type of mucus, sperm can stay healthy and able to fertilize an egg for up to five days! That means a woman can have intercourse on Monday and, if fertile mucus is present, the sperm can be waiting in the reproductive

system to fertilize an egg—even if it isn't released from the ovary until Friday! *The fact that sperm may be able to fertilize the egg up to five days after intercourse is important to remember for the successful use of natural family planning.*

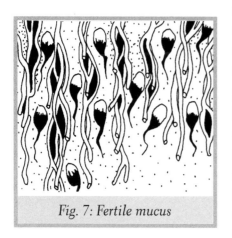

Fig. 7: Fertile mucus

Fertile cervical mucus also helps filter out unhealthy sperm. It contains channels that form "superhighways" that vibrate, helping to push the sperm up into the uterus. These channels are too narrow for some defective, unusually shaped, and larger-than-normal sperm to swim through.

7. Estrogen produces a change in the position of the uterus, causing the cervix to move upward in the vaginal canal. Estrogen also causes the cervix to soften and its opening to widen. All of these changes help sperm to travel easily into the uterus. The changes in both the mucus and the cervix can be observed by the woman, enabling her to determine her days of fertility. *Cervical mucus and changes in the cervix are two main fertility signs used to achieve or prevent a pregnancy.* For more information on these fertility signs, see the next chapter.

8. Once the egg has reached a certain level of maturity and the ovary has made enough estrogen, ovulation will occur. Ovulation is the process of the egg leaving the ovary. After this happens, the egg enters the fallopian tube.

9. As soon as ovulation has happened, the follicle goes through a major change. It becomes an entirely different structure that is yellow in color. When this happens, it is called the **corpus luteum** (Latin for "yellow body"). The corpus luteum produces

estrogen and large amounts of **progesterone**—the second major female hormone.

10. Once ovulation has taken place, progesterone controls the remainder of the fertility cycle. One of its jobs is to change the lining of the uterus so that within five to seven days after ovulation, the uterine lining is completely prepared to receive a fertilized egg.

11. A large amount of progesterone helps stop the ovaries from releasing more eggs. This means that once ovulation occurs, it will not happen again later in that same fertility cycle. Occasionally a second (and, rarely, a third or fourth) egg will be released, but if that happens, it will be within 24 hours after the release of the first egg. This explains the reason for non-identical or fraternal twins. About 1 percent of all babies born in the United States are nonidentical twins.

    After one or perhaps two eggs are released, no more will be released during the cycle. Since there are no more eggs released, there is no further chance of pregnancy. This is another important factor to remember in using fertility signs to prevent pregnancy.

12. Progesterone also causes the production of **infertile cervical mucus.** This type of mucus is made by the cervix for only one reason... to help protect a pregnancy! As strange as this many seem, even when an egg and sperm meet, the woman's body doesn't know about it

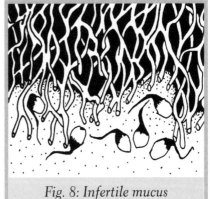

Fig. 8: Infertile mucus

for several days. However, what is amazing is that during and shortly after ovulation, the cervix and mucus automatically go through changes to help protect a pregnancy whether or not it has happened! The cervix produces infertile mucus, a protective type of mucus that helps block the opening of the cervix. If a woman does become pregnant, this type of mucus must be in the cervix for an extremely important reason. It makes it difficult for bacteria, viruses, and other substances to live and travel through the cervix and into the uterus where they could harm a pregnancy. This protective mucus is also harmful to sperm. Sperm don't like it, they are not able to live in it for more than a short period of time, and they cannot travel through it. In fact, infertile mucus has been called the best natural spermicide around!

13. As soon as ovulation takes place, the cervix becomes firm and begins to lower in the vaginal canal, and the opening closes. These changes help reduce the chances that sperm or any other foreign matter will get into the uterus and harm a pregnancy, should one have occurred.

   The special changes in the mucus and cervix that occur after ovulation can be used to determine when the fertile days have ended and the infertile days after ovulation have started. You will learn about these methods in later chapters.

We have introduced one major fertility sign that can be used to determine which days are fertile and infertile—mucus. Now it is time to learn more about another major fertility sign—basal body temperature (BBT), or the temperature of the body at rest. This invaluable sign can be used, with or without observing mucus changes, to determine when the fertile days end and the infertile days after ovulation begin.

Shortly before, during, or shortly after ovulation, a woman's body temperature usually rises noticeably from about three-tenths of a degree to one full degree Fahrenheit (0.3°F–1.0°F) higher than it had been up to that point. This happens, in part, because progesterone is a heat-producing hormone. Once the temperature has risen, it will remain high for twelve to sixteen days. It begins to lower shortly before or

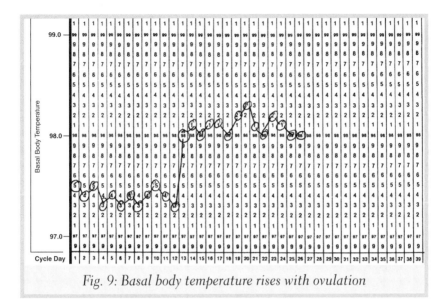

Fig. 9: Basal body temperature rises with ovulation

during the time menstrual bleeding begins again. This is because the corpus luteum produces progesterone for several days, keeping the uterine lining in place long enough for a fertilized egg to travel to it and become attached to the lining.

If the corpus luteum doesn't work well and progesterone isn't made in the right amount, the lining of the uterus can change and allow menstrual bleeding to begin too soon. Even if an egg and sperm were to meet, if menstrual bleeding began before the fertilized egg could get to the uterine lining, it would not have a place to attach and grow. This would mean that the pregnancy could not continue. This can cause fertility problems for the woman.

If pregnancy doesn't occur, the corpus luteum receives a message from the pituitary gland that it is no longer needed at that point and so it stops making estrogen and progesterone. Since these hormones are no longer present in the quantity needed to keep the uterine lining in place, the lining begins to change, allowing menstrual bleeding to take place. When this happens, a new cycle has begun.

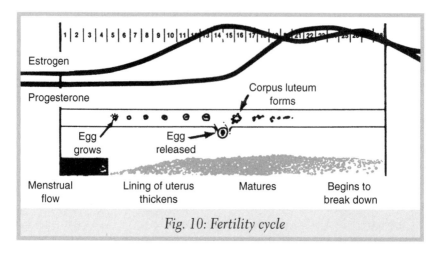

Estrogen

Progesterone

Corpus luteum forms

Egg grows

Egg released

Menstrual flow

Lining of uterus thickens

Matures

Begins to break down

Fig. 10: Fertility cycle

The changes in the amounts of estrogen and progesterone throughout a fertility cycle cause amazing changes to occur within the woman's body. Before ovulation, rising levels of estrogen are responsible for making the changes in the mucus and the cervix that allow sperm to travel into a woman's reproductive system and meet with the egg. The lining of the uterus is also changing to prepare for the possibility of pregnancy. After ovulation, rising levels of progesterone are responsible for making the changes in the mucus and cervix that help protect a pregnancy. The lining continues to prepare for the possibility of pregnancy. The changing hormone levels also cause obvious changes in cervical mucus and basal body temperature that a woman can observe to determine where she is in her cycle. This knowledge can help her time intercourse in order to prevent or achieve a pregnancy.

Menstruation Through History

It took centuries for the medical community to develop the technology and understanding to discover ovulation and the ways in which a woman's body changes to enable her to become pregnant. Until this happened, menstrual bleeding was the only aspect of a woman's fertility that was known, simply because it could be easily seen. Over four hundred years ago, menstrual bleeding was given the name **menses** from the Latin word for "monthly." Over time, it has been called many different names, such as "period," "friend," "curse," "falling off the roof," and "being on the rag." Throughout history and even today, menstrual bleeding has been thought of more often as a "curse" than a "friend"! There are many reasons for this. During ancient times, bleeding was associated with the life process. People believed that life went on as long as the blood stayed in the body. To bleed meant to be injured and frequently to die. Therefore, for a woman to bleed and not be hurt was an unexplained mystery. Almost every religion and culture has formed beliefs about this mystery of women, often viewing it in a negative way. Menstruating women were thought to be possessed either by evil or by good spirits. In some prehistoric cultures women were regarded as goddesses. They were felt to possess supernatural powers. If women could control the life force, they could also control the weather, the growth of crops, birth, and death.

This powerful, godlike role given to women was soon turned upside down. As soon as the early civilizations realized women who continued menstruating were not helping to increase the population, menstruation became a "curse." Women were said to be possessed by the devil and were called witches. When they were menstruating, they were considered to be dangerous to men. In fact, women were blamed for just about everything. If crops died, milk curdled, meat spoiled, or a tornado or hurricane came along, guess who was blamed? In some cultures, women had to live in special places away from their homes during menstruation. This was to protect everyone from harm, since the gaze of a menstruating woman was said to soften men's bones and prevent them from fighting well during a battle!

Obviously this attitude about menstruation was based upon ignorance and fear. Many women today still feel the effects of this history. Many women and men feel that menstruation is unclean, instead of viewing it as the end of one fertility cycle and the beginning of the next—nothing more, nothing less.

TO REVIEW

During the first part of the fertility cycle, the egg develops and the cervix rises, softens, opens, and produces fertile mucus. These changes keep the sperm alive and healthy and allow them to travel to the egg. They can also help a woman identify the days before ovulation when she can and cannot become pregnant and when her fertile time before ovulation begins. The basal body temperature is usually low during this time.

Once the egg leaves its follicle, the cervix closes and infertile mucus is produced. These changes help to protect a pregnancy if it should occur. The basal body temperature rises. All of these changes help a woman identify when her fertile time has ended and her infertile time after ovulation has begun.

YOUR NOTES

5

Your Fertility Signs

It's important to learn all you can about your fertility cycle so that you are able to use natural family planning or the fertility awareness method as effectively as possible. *Awareness is important.* In this section we emphasize a special kind of awareness—**fertility awareness:** learning about your fertility signs and the way in which you can observe their changing patterns during your fertility cycles.

The two most important fertility signs are:

❖ cervical mucus

❖ basal body temperature

Another major fertility sign that can be observed is the cervix.

Cervical Mucus Changes

Cervical mucus is normal, healthy, and an important aspect of your fertility. As we have discussed previously, you can use mucus changes to know when you can and cannot become pregnant by learning to recognize the qualities of fertile and infertile mucus.

If you are going to use your mucus to determine when your fertile and infertile days begin and end, you will need to learn about the different mucus changes you can experience and the ways in which you will look for these changes. When you have this information and note the changes you observe on your fertility awareness chart, you are then able to apply simple instructions that will enable you to accurately know which days you can and cannot become pregnant.

Remember: Fertile mucus helps a woman become pregnant; infertile mucus prevents pregnancy.

Both fertile and infertile mucus have their own special:

❖ color

❖ quantity

❖ feel

Both fertile and infertile mucus also cause the vaginal area (the area in and around the vaginal opening and the vaginal lips) to have its own special feelings, or what are known as "vaginal sensations." These are not felt by touching the vaginal area. Instead, these are sensations that a woman observes by thinking about them. A woman must think to herself: "Do my vaginal lips and/or the area around my vaginal opening feel wet? Do I feel a slipperiness or lubrication type of feeling?" Some women are already familiar with this wet, lubricated feeling during some of the days of their fertility cycle but do not realize it is a reflection of their fertility and the type of cervical mucus being produced. They may think the wetness is caused by a vaginal infection or by neglecting to wash the vaginal area well enough, or for some other unknown reason.

It is the combination of cervical mucus and vaginal sensations that provide a woman with the information she needs to use NFP. When we discuss the cervical mucus pattern below, please try to imagine the quality of vaginal sensations you might feel when you are producing a particular type of mucus. This will serve as a form of exercise to help you develop awareness of vaginal sensations.

The Different Cervical Mucus Patterns

The number of days a woman has infertile and fertile types of mucus can vary from fertility cycle to fertility cycle. The characteristics of the mucus can also vary to some degree, yet the basic mucus pattern for most women is… DRY … to WET … to DRY. This means that early in the fertility cycle and after menstrual bleeding ends, a woman can expect to experience days in which there is no wet mucus. Often she won't be able to see or feel any kind of mucus on these days. (Vaginal sensations are usually dry.) Alternatively, sometimes she will see mucus, but it does not feel wet. This type is called "non-wet" mucus. (Vaginal sensations are dry or sticky feeling.) Eventually, as the time of ovulation nears, the mucus will become wet, slippery, and stretchy. There may even be a small amount of blood mixed in with the slippery, wet mucus. (Vaginal sensations are wet.) After ovulation, the mucus loses its wet, slippery, and stretchy qualities. (Vaginal sensations are sticky or dry.) The pattern we've just described is very basic and a reflection of rising and falling levels of hormones that occur as the egg is growing and after the egg has come out of the ovary.

Before we describe a few examples of typical mucus patterns, it is important to know how to observe mucus.

A Few Words on Cervical Mucus Observation

Before we describe the actual steps to mucus checking, we would like to offer some information that, should you need it, might serve as encouragement for you as you are learning about your mucus changes.

1. Mucus observations are not something you have to do every day of your life for as long as you use NFP or FAM. They begin when menstrual bleeding ends and are continued for a few to several days, depending upon the length of your fertility cycles. You can stop checking your mucus for the remainder of the menstrual cycle after you have applied information to your mucus changes that let you know you are past ovulation and can no longer become pregnant.

2. You may become comfortable enough to use your mucus changes to prevent pregnancy after you have carefully observed them for 2 to 4 weeks. Some women find their mucus pattern very easy to learn and are confident using it for pregnancy prevention within a short period of time.

3. Some women ask, "How will I know the difference between wet and non-wet mucus?" When you observe your mucus, you need to give yourself the opportunity to experience the different types of changes so that you can compare them to each other. When you do this, the difference between wet mucus and non-wet mucus is usually quite obvious.

4. The only kind of mucus observation we recommend is called **external checking**, or checking for mucus at the vaginal opening. The reason for this is that all of the best research about NFP has been performed using external checking. If you insert a finger into the vagina to get a sample of mucus, you can become confused trying to determine the difference between normal vaginal discharge and cervical mucus. The last thing you want when you are learning all this great, but new information, is to feel confused!

5. Normal vaginal moisture you might experience throughout the day, including perspiration, is absorbed by toilet tissue. Mucus stays on top of the toilet tissue.

Directions for Mucus and Vaginal Sensations

Begin mucus observations when menstrual bleeding stops or decreases to the point that you can accurately check mucus, such as when you are only spotting a little bit of blood. On the days you need to observe your mucus changes, it is important to begin doing so at some point soon after you awaken and before you bathe and go to the bathroom. Before making the actual mucus observation, ask yourself this question: "Does the area around the outside of my vaginal opening and in the vaginal opening **feel** wet and/or slippery or does it feel dry or sticky?" When we use the word "feel," we don't mean you will touch the area, but instead, you will **think** about it. It's like thinking "Am I cold or hot?" "Is my skin wet or dry?" You can answer these questions without touching your body, simply by being aware of the physical changes you are experiencing. This may sound strange when it comes to the vagina, but it's true! When you think about the way in which the vaginal area feels, you are learning about your vaginal sensations or vaginal feelings. These are the sensations that are important to learn, and you have probably noticed them before as a result of different circumstances. For example, if you had intercourse and semen was in your vagina, it most likely felt wet and slippery up to several hours after intercourse. You didn't have to touch your vaginal area, you knew it by the sensation of wetness. A vaginal medication or spermicide can make the vaginal area feel wet or sticky. Being sexually aroused creates a wet feeling in the vaginal area. Perspiration can also make the vaginal area feel wet. Many women state that they are aware of a wet feeling shortly before their period begins and often find themselves going to the bathroom to see if they have begun menstruating.

Vaginal sensations are important to understand because they can serve as signals as to the type of mucus being produced. For example, if the cervix is producing wet mucus, it will make the outside of the vagina feel wet. As ovulation approaches and mucus becomes wet, it develops slippery, stretchy characteristics that make the vaginal area feel slippery and lubricated. The vaginal area can even feel slightly swollen, causing a woman to feel a sense of fullness and perhaps a feeling of greater sensitivity. Mucus that doesn't have a wet consistency and that is sometimes described as sticky, pasty, and crumbly will make the outside of the vagina feel dry or sticky. When mucus is not being produced, the outside of the vagina usually feels dry as well.

Please remember, vaginal sensations are not experienced by touching the vaginal area with the fingers. They are feelings a woman mentally "tunes in to." While walking, sitting, or lying down, a woman needs to ask herself: "Does my vaginal area feel wet or dry? Does it feel slippery, full, or swollen?" Through continuous practice, assessing vaginal sensations becomes easier and easier. In fact, some women become so experienced with their vaginal sensations that they know which type of mucus they are producing without even using the mucus checking technique described below. Even if you reach this level of experience, we still strongly suggest that you continue checking mucus regularly. Combining knowledge of vaginal sensations and cervical mucus is the best choice when using this information to prevent pregnancy.

Once you have decided how the outside of the vagina feels, the next step is to look at the mucus. There are three steps to doing this:

1. Take a piece of folded white toilet tissue and wipe the outside of the vaginal opening.

2. Next, look at the toilet tissue and answer these questions:
   - Is there any mucus on the toilet tissue?
   - If so, what color is it?
   - How much mucus is on the toilet tissue?
3. Then determine how the mucus feels.
   - Take a sample of the mucus between two fingers to determine how it feels.
   - Part the fingers slowly to see if the mucus stretches or just forms little peaks.
   - Does the mucus feel sticky, pasty, and crumbly, or does it feel wet? Does it feel stretchy and slippery?

Your cervical mucus should be checked a few times during the day because mucus can change at different times. For example, it can be pasty and sticky in the morning and afternoon, but by nighttime it can be wet and stretchy. The more often you check your mucus, the better. Many women find it convenient to check their cervical mucus whenever they use the bathroom.

Kegel Exercises

No doubt there have been occasions when you needed to use the bathroom and there was no bathroom in sight. To prevent an accident, you tightly squeezed the muscles "down there" to prevent the flow of urine. These muscles that surround the vagina are called the pubococcygeal (PC) muscles. Kegel exercises involve the tightening and relaxing of these PC muscles. It is good to do them regularly because they help keep the muscles strong which, in turn, helps keep the bladder in place so that urinary problems may be prevented as women become older.

The exercises are easy to do and can be performed anywhere without anyone knowing you're doing them! To perform Kegel exercises, squeeze your vaginal opening as tight as you can, pretending you are stopping the flow of urine. This motion causes the muscles to contract. Hold the squeeze for five seconds, then relax the muscles. Repeat the tightening and relaxing of the muscles at least ten times a few times a

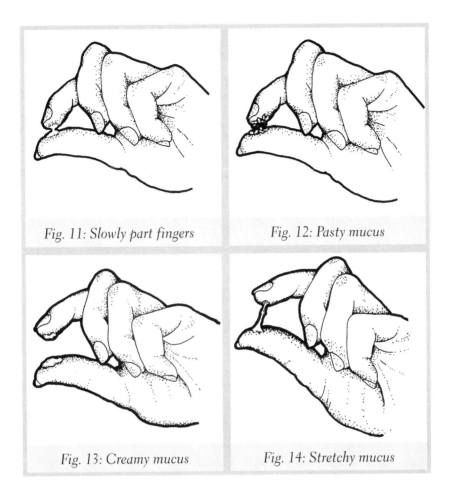

Fig. 11: *Slowly part fingers*

Fig. 12: *Pasty mucus*

Fig. 13: *Creamy mucus*

Fig. 14: *Stretchy mucus*

day. Not only is this a healthy exercise to do, and one that some women feel helps to increase sexual pleasure for themselves and their partner, but it may also help push any mucus at the cervix down to the vaginal opening. Because of this, you may want to perform the exercise before you check for mucus.

Other excellent times to check cervical mucus are following physical exercise or bowel movements. As with the Kegel exercise, these activities can cause the mucus to travel down to the vaginal opening. In fact, if you are having difficulty seeing mucus on days you think you should be seeing it, make a point to check for mucus after any type of exercise, Kegel exercises, and a bowel movement.

Three Typical Mucus Patterns

Now that you know how to check your mucus and vaginal sensations, let's look at examples of the three typical mucus patterns that can occur after menstrual bleeding has ended.

PATTERN NUMBER 1. After menstrual bleeding ends, you may not see mucus for one to a few days, and your vaginal sensations may be dry. There is absolutely no wet or slippery feeling around the vaginal lips and vaginal opening. Days without any mucus and dry vaginal sensations are called "dry days." Some women notice this dryness toward the end of their menstrual flow. When removing a tampon, they experience discomfort because there is so little moisture in the vaginal area from a lack of cervical mucus. Some women notice intercourse is not as comfortable for them during these dry days. Though they feel sexually aroused and have vaginal lubrication, they still may not feel as comfortable as compared to days when wet mucus is being made and mixes with the wetness created by sexual arousal.

A woman who has a few to several dry days before her fertile days begin is experiencing her **basic infertile pattern** (BIP) or the way in which her body signals her that she is experiencing an infertile time. This makes sense because, as you know, fertile mucus is produced as ovulation nears and is needed for sperm life and travel. Therefore, the chances of anyone becoming pregnant from having intercourse on dry days is highly unlikely!

PATTERN NUMBER 2. When the menstrual flow ends, you may start to produce mucus right away. This is more common for women who have short fertility cycles, such as those that are less than 26 days long. The mucus is often a kind that doesn't feel wet but instead feels sticky, pasty, or crumbly and can look whitish-yellow on your underwear. It is not a wet-feeling mucus. It doesn't stretch. It may form very small peaks on the finger as you are trying to stretch it. Since it contains very little moisture, it causes the vaginal area to feel dry or sticky.

PATTERN NUMBER 3. When the menstrual flow ends, you may produce a mucus right away that feels wet and looks creamy and white. It doesn't feel slippery yet, and it may stretch a very small amount or may not stretch at all. This type of mucus often causes a wet feeling around the vaginal opening.

To review these patterns, once the menstrual flow ends, you may experience the following:

1. A dry feeling at the opening of the vagina, with no mucus present.

2. A dry or sticky feeling at the opening of the vagina, with sticky, pasty, crumbly mucus.

3. A wet feeling at the opening of the vagina with a wet-feeling mucus that is often creamy.

Changes in Mucus as Ovulation Approaches

Regardless of whether you are dry or you begin to produce non-wet or wet mucus after the menstrual flow ends, women who are ovulating experience the same change as ovulation approaches. This change is the production of increasingly wetter mucus. Remember that the closer the approach of ovulation, the wetter the mucus becomes. This is due to the fact that as ovulation approaches, more estrogen is made because the egg is getting ready to leave the ovary. The rising level of estrogen causes glands in the cervix to produce the wetter mucus.

In addition, the amount of mucus can increase, and it usually becomes clear and can be opaque. It may even be pink from the slight amount of blood that can normally come out of the uterus. It can be stretched between two fingers (Figure 14) This type of mucus has the appearance and texture of raw egg white. Known as **spinnbarkeit** (pronounced spin-bar-kite), it can look like the shimmering strands of a spider web. Wet, slippery, lubricating mucus causes a wet, slippery, lubricated feeling around your vaginal lips and at the opening of your vagina, along with an increase of wet mucus on your underwear. Some women have misunderstood this wet mucus, considering it to be the sign of a vaginal infection. This is not so!

During the time when your mucus is at its wettest and most slippery and your vaginal sensations are slippery and lubricated with perhaps a sense of fullness or slight swollen feeling, your estrogen level has reached its highest point in the fertility cycle. Does this mean that the day when the mucus is most wet, slippery, and stretchy is the exact day of ovulation? Not necessarily. It could be, but ovulation could have taken place already, or could be about to occur within a day or so. There are different reports as to when ovulation occurs in relation to certain mucus changes. Researchers have presented different opinions and theories as to when a woman is most fertile according to her mucus changes. Determining the day of greatest fertility is difficult if not impossible to accomplish—either through home tests or through a medical facility. This is also true when attempting to determine the exact time of ovulation. However, this does not matter when it comes to NFP. NFP is based on knowing when the fertile days begin and end. At some point during these days, ovulation will take place. Knowing the exact day of ovulation is completely unnecessary when using NFP, regardless of whether you are using it to prevent or achieve pregnancy. Please think "fertile time" as opposed to "the day of ovulation." Rather than focusing on the exact time of ovulation, think about the most fertile versus the less fertile days. When using NFP for pregnancy prevention, you can imagine how focusing on a particular day or two could cause needless anxiety and perhaps an unplanned pregnancy. The fact is, a little fertile mucus can get a woman "a little pregnant!" The beauty of NFP is that it is not dependent on a particular day but on the number of days of a cycle that have been clearly shown to be fertile.

You know that soon after ovulation, the mucus must become the type that helps to protect a pregnancy. This infertile type of mucus is produced by rising levels of progesterone that occur right after ovulation. As progesterone levels rise, the wet feeling at the outside of the vaginal opening disappears, and the mucus becomes sticky or pasty, or mucus won't be seen at all. Some women have a constant dry feeling at the outside of the vagina for the remainder of their fertility cycle. Other women continue to have pasty mucus and sticky or dry vaginal feelings until their next fertility cycle begins. A couple of days before menstrual bleeding starts, some women notice a wet discharge and wet feeling at the outside of the vaginal opening. Although the mucus feels wet, it is not fertile mucus. It is fluid from the lining of the uterus that flows out of the vagina prior to the start of menstrual bleeding.

Many women notice these normal mucus changes throughout their fertility cycles—the wet and dry feelings, the increase and decrease in vaginal secretions, and the color changes—yet have never associated these changes with their fertility patterns.

> *Cervical mucus changes and vaginal feelings (or sensations) are the main fertility signs, which enable a woman to know when her fertile days have started—at some point during the fertile days, ovulation will take place. Cervical mucus and vaginal feelings can also be used to know when the fertile days have ended.*

WARNING! The change from the sticky, pasty, crumbly infertile type of mucus to the wet, fertile type of mucus can be difficult to see and feel when you are first learning about your mucus changes. Therefore, you may miss detecting a small amount of fertile mucus mixed with infertile mucus. In addition, you might see only infertile mucus on the toilet tissue at a time when slippery, stretchy, and wet fertile mucus is already being produced up in the cervix. It may take a day or so for this mucus to travel to the vaginal opening where it can be seen. Therefore, it is extremely important to know that when preventing pregnancy, after the menstrual bleeding ends, *any type of mucus that appears before ovulation is considered potentially fertile.*

This means that if unprotected intercourse takes place when any type of mucus is seen before ovulation, a pregnancy may result.

A Special Note about Cervical Mucus

It is important to remember that certain factors can affect the cervical mucus, preventing the accurate observations needed to apply the mucus rules successfully. (You will learn about the mucus rules in Chapters 9 and 10. These factors are

1. *Douching*, which removes most cervical mucus from the vaginal canal. Douching does not remove *all* of the mucus in the vagina nor can it remove much that is up in the cervix, which is why this is not a successful method of birth control. However, it can remove enough of the mucus to make cervical mucus observations inaccurate.

2. *Semen* in the vaginal canal after intercourse. The semen mixes with cervical mucus, making accurate observation of mucus very difficult if not impossible.

3. *Sexual arousal*, which causes moisture to form in the vaginal canal, making it difficult to determine when mucus is present. You should wait until the wet feeling from sexual arousal is gone before checking for cervical mucus.

4. *Spermicidal agents* (creams, jellies, suppositories, film, and foams), which remain in the vagina for a day or more after their use. You should not use them if you want to observe your mucus as accurately as possible.

5. A *vaginal infection and vaginal medication*, which can prevent accurate observation of cervical mucus. Strategies for handling these situations are discussed in Chapter 10.

Basal Body Temperature

The second major fertility sign is your basal body temperature (BBT), or the temperature of the body after you have rested for several hours. As hormone levels change over the course of the fertility cycle, the BBT changes, too. It is an excellent signal of when the fertile days end and the infertile days after ovulation begin. The BBT is often at a low level when menstrual bleeding begins. Sometimes, however, it can be as high or almost as high as it was after ovulation during the previous cycle. In other words, it may take a few days during menstrual bleeding for the BBT to return to a low level. Once this happens, it will stay low for several days. It then usually makes an obvious rise of 0.3°F to 1.0°F (0.15–0.5°C)

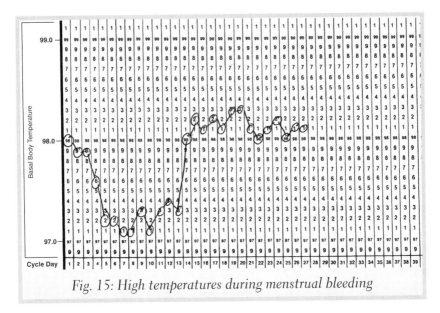

Fig. 15: High temperatures during menstrual bleeding

higher than it had been up to that point (Figure 15). The rise usually occurs shortly before, during, or shortly after ovulation.

The BBT may not always rise in an extremely obvious way near the time of ovulation. Instead, it may rise slowly, creating its own unique pattern. When charted, this pattern may resemble stair steps (Figure 16). The BBT will rise steadily and eventually go up to its highest point. Different patterns can be experienced, but they all have in common one important fact. The BBT will be low for a few to several days, and then it will be higher for several days once ovulation has taken place.

Basal Body Temperature Observation

As with our discussion about cervical mucus observation, we would like to offer some information about BBT observations that might be helpful to you as you are learning about this fertility sign.

1. Basal body temperature does not need to taken every day while you are using fertility signs for family planning. We recommend taking it every day for one complete fertility cycle to have the experience of seeing your complete BBT pattern. However, once you get used to observing your BBT, you can

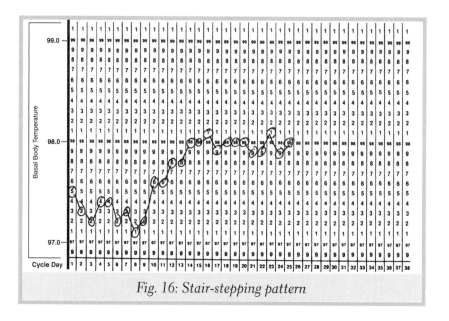

Fig. 16: Stair-stepping pattern

begin to take it starting on the last day of your period and continue until it changes in a way that lets you know ovulation has
passed. At that point, you can put the thermometer away for
the rest of the cycle.

2. Basal body temperature can usually be used during the first
   cycle it is observed to determine when the infertile days after
   ovulation have started.

3. Ideally, you should use a glass basal body temperature
   thermometer. This is a special thermometer that is marked in
   measurements of 0.1°F ($^1/_{10}$ of a degree Fahrenheit) or 0.05°C
   ($^1/_{20}$ of a degree Centigrade), allowing greater accuracy in mea-
   suring basal body temperature changes. Fever thermometers
   are usually marked in measurements of 0.2°F ($^2/_{10}$ of a degree
   Fahrenheit). Since the basal body temperature thermometer
   can provide a more accurate reading, you may achieve better
   results by using one. However, many stores are now selling
   small digital basal body temperature thermometers, that are
   more durable, take readings quickly, and hold the last tempera-

ture in memory until the next use. Keep in mind, though, that the majority of digital thermometers are not developed to record BBT, and that their accuracy and reliability as they relate to NFP have not yet been determined.

4. The temperature can be taken orally, vaginally, or rectally. Vaginal and rectal temperatures can be up to one full degree Fahrenheit higher than oral temperatures. Therefore, you should use the same method to take the temperature consistently throughout a particular cycle. For example, if you begin taking your temperature orally, it is important to continue taking it orally for the remainder of that cycle. If you want or need to take the BBT some other way, it is best to start doing this with the next cycle.

5. Some people have asked whether using a digital thermometer or taking the temperature in the ear, under the arm, or using the bands placed on the forehead to monitor temperature works as well as a glass thermometer. Taking the temperature anywhere besides the mouth, rectum, or vagina is not advisable. Using other parts of the body to take the BBT has not been studied for use with NFP and may not be accurate. The majority of digital thermometers are designed for monitoring fever. Are they as reliable as a glass thermometer for everyone? This is not known. Some women state they experience an accurate BBT pattern using a digital thermometer. However, all the controlled research on using BBT for pregnancy prevention has been conducted using glass thermometers. There have been no studies done to prove that digital thermometers are reliable for everyone for this purpose. If you want to use a digital thermometer because it is more convenient, we urge you to take your temperature with a glass thermometer and a digital thermometer for one or two complete cycles and compare the temperatures. If they are the same or give you the same beginning time for the infertile phase, the digital thermometer is probably fine for you to use.

The Steps for Taking Your BBT

This is how you take your basal body temperature:

1. Take your temperature as soon as you awaken, before you get out of bed or engage in any kind of activity, such as eating, drinking, or smoking.

2. Take your temperature either orally (under your tongue), rectally (in your rectum), or vaginally (in your vagina) for five minutes. Since it is important to be consistent, use the same method each time you take your temperature.

   Many women find that taking their temperature orally is most convenient. However, sinus or breathing problems may require that you take your temperature vaginally or rectally.

   It must be remembered that temperatures taken vaginally and rectally are about 1°F or 0.5°C higher than oral temperatures. Therefore, taking your temperature rectally or vaginally one day and orally another day may not provide an accurate account of the temperature pattern.

   If for some reason you have to take your temperature differently one day, be sure to make a note of this on your fertility awareness chart.

3. Once the five minutes are up, read the thermometer and record your temperature on the chart. If you feel like going back to sleep after taking your temperature, put the thermometer in a safe place and read the thermometer later. Be careful not to place it near a heater, a lamp, or by a window, since the reading could easily be affected by the heat.

4. Once the BBT is recorded, the mercury in the thermometer should be shaken down and the thermometer placed safely in its case, available for use the next day.

5. Take your BBT at about the same time every day. This guarantees a more accurate temperature pattern throughout

the fertility cycle. However, if you oversleep one day or need to awaken earlier than usual another day, take your BBT when you wake up and record it. Note the different time you took the BBT on your fertility awareness chart. An occasional early or late temperature will probably not affect your ability to use the temperature for family planning.

6. When the BBT is recorded daily, it is important to make note of anything that may cause the temperature to be unusual. For example, taking the temperature in a different manner than usual, drinking alcoholic beverages the night before, taking a medication or a drug, awakening later or earlier than usual, or a restless night's sleep may make the temperature abnormally high or low. These events may not cause a change, but as long as they have been recorded, if they do affect your temperature, you can make adjustments for them.

7. If the mercury in the thermometer is between two lines, the lower of the two temperatures is recorded. For example, if the mercury reads between 97.1°F and 97.2°F, the 97.1°F reading is recorded as the temperature for the day.

8. Regardless of how the temperature is taken, you should try not to fall asleep with the thermometer in place. Rolling over may break it. The thermometer could also fall out of place, causing an inaccurate reading for the day.

Using the BBT Thermometer

Place the rounded mercury end of the thermometer under your tongue. Try to put it in the same area each day since some areas of the mouth are warmer than others. Keep your lips closed over the thermometer

or

Place the first half-inch of the thermometer in the rectum (Putting Vaseline or an oil on the tip of the thermometer makes inserting a rectal thermometer more comfortable)

or

Place the first half-inch of the thermometer into the vaginal opening (Do not use any type of lubrication—oil or jelly—since these can affect mucus observations)

REVIEW

✤ Use a basal body temperature thermometer.

✤ Take your temperature just after you wake up.

✤ Do not engage in any activity before you take your temperature—no smoking, eating, drinking, or sexual activity.

✤ Take your temperature at the same time each day.

✤ Keep the thermometer in place for five minutes.

These temperature-taking instructions should be followed as closely as possible. If an unexpected situation occurs—you need to go to the bathroom, care for a child, or answer a phone call—you should take your temperature as soon as you are able to.

Remember, your BBT is your body temperature at rest, unaffected by activity—drinking, smoking, eating, etc. For the woman who works evenings or nights, the temperature should be taken when she normally wakes up.

For some women, the basal body temperature is difficult to observe because it requires awakening at about the same time every day. On the other hand, some women find that taking their temperature is not difficult, and it is a good time to relax and plan the day's activities. Some women have said that the process has helped them establish a routine of getting up a little earlier so that they have time for breakfast or an exercise routine they have wanted to enjoy.

If you are unable to take your temperature upon awakening and at the same time, you can try this: Take your temperature at the same time every night between 8:00 P.M. and midnight, after one hour of relaxing (putting your feet up and taking it easy).

This way of taking the BBT works well for some women but doesn't work for others.

You can also try the following way to take your BBT. Awaken around the same time every day and go to the bathroom. Urinate into a plastic or paper cup. (Metal or glass cups may be too cold and may change the temperature of the urine.) Place the thermometer in the urine with the mercury facing the bottom of the glass. Urine is basically the same temperature as the body at rest. Because of this, some women have found that when a thermometer is left in a cup with their urine for 5 minutes, the temperature of the urine is an accurate measure of their BBT.

The Basic BBT Pattern

As we have discussed, when your menstrual period starts, your BBT will usually be in a low range. This range could be one of 96.0°F to 97.4°F (or 35.4°C to 36.8°C). Some women experience BBTs that go above this range. If this happens to you, it is not a problem. It is only a reflection of the effect of the progesterone from the previous cycle (the hormone causes body temperature to rise). If this happens, the BBT will usually drop down to its low level by the time the menstrual flow ends, and will remain low until around the time of ovulation.

The key with the BBT pattern is that shortly before, during, or shortly after ovulation, the BBT will rise to an obviously higher level, usually from 0.3°F to 1.0°F (0.15°C to 0.5°C) greater than the level of the BBT readings from at least a few days prior to this rise in temperature.

After the BBT rises, it should remain in a high range for about twelve to sixteen days. Menstrual bleeding usually occurs when the temperature begins to fall. If your basal body temperature remains high longer than 20 days and sexual intercourse occurred during a fertile time, this can be a reliable sign of pregnancy.

Is it correct to say that ovulation takes place the day before the temperature rise? NO! It often does, but it can also take place up to a few days before the rise, the day of the temperature rise, or the day after the rise. It doesn't actually matter exactly when ovulation takes place, because once the BBT has risen and remained elevated for 3 days, you have proof that the egg has been released and is no longer around to meet with sperm. When this has happened, pregnancy is not possible for the remainder of the cycle.

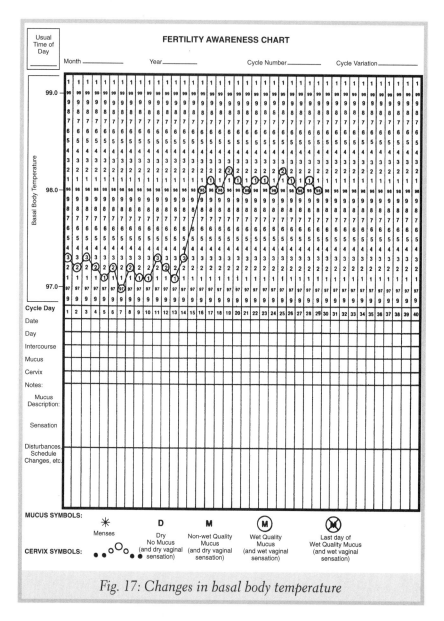

Fig. 17: Changes in basal body temperature

Changes in the Cervix

Another fertility sign some women choose to monitor is the cervix. Although cervical changes do not have to be observed to determine days of fertility and infertility, they can provide additional information about a woman's fertility pattern.

As you know, when ovulation approaches, mucus becomes fertile to help keep sperm healthy and allow them to travel easily up into the cervix. And as previously mentioned, the opening of the cervix also changes during ovulation by widening a litle bit to help sperm travel. When we say "a litle bit" we mean that it only becomes about as wide as the tip of your little or index finger. This helps sperm get up into the uterus. The cervical opening also becomes this wide during menstruation, to let blood flow out of the uterus (see Figure 18, "Changes in the cervix").

After menstruation ends, the opening is closed. Then it opens around the time of ovulation. After ovulation, the opening closes again. A closed cervical opening after ovulation, in combination with infertile cervical mucus, helps protect against pregnancy.

All of this means that the basic pattern of changes in the cervical opening is: closed after menstrual bleeding ends, opened as ovulation nears, and then closed again after ovulation.

During the menstrual period, the cervix is low in the vaginal canal and usually easy to reach with a finger. The area surrounding its opening is soft.

When the period ends, the cervix is still usually easy to feel. If you touch it with your finger, you can feel that your cervix is closer to your vaginal opening and it feels firm, like the tip of a nose or a small rubber ball, and the opening is closed.

As ovulation approaches, the rising estrogen levels cause the cervix to move away from the vaginal opening. Therefore, you may have to insert a finger further into the vagina to feel it. Also, the cervical opening begins to widen and the area surrounding it softens. The rising and opening of the cervix helps sperm travel into the uterus.

After ovulation, the rising progesterone level causes the cervix once again to lower in the vaginal canal and become easier to reach. The cervical opening becomes smaller or closes and the area around it becomes firmer. These changes help prevent sperm from entering the uterus.

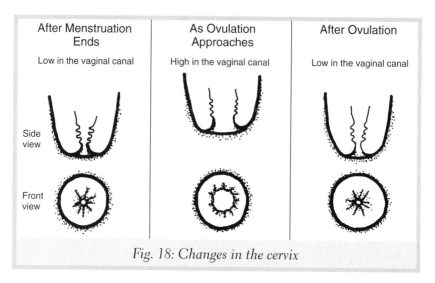

Fig. 18: Changes in the cervix

Is it correct to say that ovulation took place when the cervix was at its highest, softest, and widest open time? Not necessarily. It may have, but changes in the cervix (as with changes in BBT and mucus) cannot be used to determine the exact time of ovulation. Changes in the cervix can tell you that the egg is preparing to leave the ovary. They can also be used as a signal that the egg has left the ovary. But they are *not* a signal of precisely when ovulation occurs.

Just as some women have noticed their changing mucus signs without connecting them to their fertility patterns, some are familiar with some aspects of their cervical changes, such as changes in the position of the cervix. For example, inserting a tampon or having intercourse in certain positions can be uncomfortable when the cervix is in its low position. Many women have experienced this but didn't know it was due to normal changes that occur during their fertility cycle.

Observing the Cervix

If you wish to observe your cervical changes, you can do this at the same time that you check your cervical mucus.

The changes in the cervix are felt by taking the following steps (see Figure 19, "Checking the cervix"):

1. Wash your hands before checking the cervix to avoid the possibility of vaginal infection.

2. Insert one or two fingers into the vaginal opening.

3. Apply gentle pressure to move the finger up the vaginal canal.

   When the finger has reached the back of the vagina, the cervix can be felt. It is smooth and round, and feels firmer than the tissue of the vagina that surrounds it.

4. As you gently but firmly feel the cervix, answer the following questions:

   - Is it easy or difficult to reach the cervix? In other words, is the cervix low or high in the vaginal canal?

   - Does the area around the cervical opening feel firm like the tip of a nose? Or does it feel soft like the lips of a mouth?

   - Does the opening feel closed, like a small dimple? Or does it feel open, like a small hole?

5. The cervix should be checked often during the day, if possible. If this is not possible, it should be checked at least once in the morning and once in the evening.

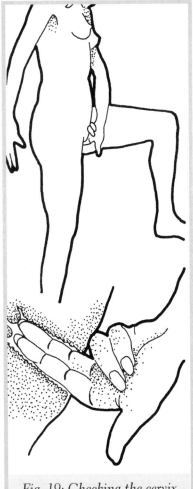

Fig. 19: Checking the cervix

6. Standing with one foot on a stool or squatting are good positions for cervical checking. The same position should be used each time the cervix is checked.

It may be difficult to learn about cervical changes if you have never seen your cervix. Therefore, you can ask your clinician to show you your cervix by using a mirror. If you are not comfortable seeing your cervix, the clinician can draw a picture of your cervix or show you a picture of a cervix.

In a woman who has not had a vaginal delivery, the closed opening can feel like a dimple; a woman who has delivered vaginally may have a cervical opening that feels irregular and somewhat opened. The shape of the cervical opening depends upon the size of the baby, the course of labor, and who delivered the baby. Sometimes, the cervix can even heal in a way that makes it look like it is divided into two parts. Also, if you have delivered children vaginally, you may have relaxed support of the uterus, making it difficult to feel the rising and lowering of the cervix.

Although the combination of cervical mucus and basal body temperature changes provides enough information to identify the fertile and infertile days accurately, some women have found observing cervical changes to be valuable in helping them determine these days.

TO REVIEW

THE MAIN FERTILITY SIGNS

* ✦ cervical mucus and vaginal feelings
* ✦ basal body temperature
* ✦ changes in the cervix

VAGINAL SENSATIONS

* ✦ How does the outside of the vaginal area feel?
  - Does it feel wet?
  - Does it feel slippery and lubricated?
  - Is there a feeling of fullness and greater sensitivity?

  – Does it feel dry?

  – Does it feel sticky?

CERVICAL MUCUS

- ❖ Collect some mucus and look at it
  – Is it yellow or white?
  – Is it clear or cloudy?
  – Is there any blood in it?
- ❖ Feel the mucus
  – Is it creamy?
  – Is it wet? Is it slippery?
  – Is it pasty or sticky?
  – Is it crumbly?
- ❖ Try to stretch the mucus between your fingers
  – Is it stretchy, or not?

CERVICAL CHANGES

- ❖ Relax and find the best position
- ❖ Feel the opening of the cervix
- ❖ Is the cervix difficult or easy to reach (high or low)?
- ❖ Is it soft or firm?
- ❖ Is it opening or closing (as compared to the way it felt the last time it was checked)?

These signs enable you to make accurate and sensible choices concerning your fertility. Remember that the fertility signs cannot be used to determine the exact day of ovulation. Instead, they are used to identify the fertile and infertile days of each fertility cycle. Knowing which days are fertile and which are infertile provides you with an excellent way of planning sexual intercourse to either achieve or prevent pregnancy.

6

Secondary Fertility Signs

Now that you know about the patterns of the major fertility signs and ways to observe them, you might be wondering if there are any other fertility signs used to help determine the fertile and infertile days. The answer is no. However, you might experience what are called secondary fertility signs, or signs that can help you better understand your body and your fertility cycle. It is important to note that not all women experience these signs—and for those who do experience them, the signs may not always be predictable. They may occur during some cycles and not during others.

Possible Secondary Fertility Signs As Ovulation Approaches

For example, as ovulation approaches, some women notice their complexion appears different, often smoother, clearer, and less oily. The reason for this is that as ovulation approaches, the body's oil-producing glands make less oil. This causes the skin and hair to become less oily and, for some women, results in a clearer complexion. Some women also find at this time their bodies begin to "hold water"—this is referred to as fluid retention. Fluid retention causes a slight bloated feeling, slight breast tenderness, and even irritability. These feelings are not as severe as those experienced premenstrually, and they usually last for only a day or two.

Some women notice an increase in energy shortly before ovulation. In fact, some women even experience a sharper sense of vision, smell, and taste as ovulation approaches.

A dull ache or pain may occur in the pelvic area shortly before, during, or shortly after ovulation. This can occur below the belly button and can travel to different areas in the lower belly, where the uterus is located. Sometimes an ache or pain can be experienced on one side of the lower belly or on both sides. This pain or ache may last a few minutes or a few days. It may travel down one or both legs and even around to the lower back. This pain may be accompanied by spotting or a light flow of blood.

Though this can be experienced with every cycle, sometimes a woman can experience it very infrequently so that when it happens, particularly if it is painful, it can be alarming to her. Sometimes this pain has been misdiagnosed as an infection in the pelvis or as appendicitis.

Around the time of ovulation, some women notice an increase in sexual feelings. Others experience no change or even a

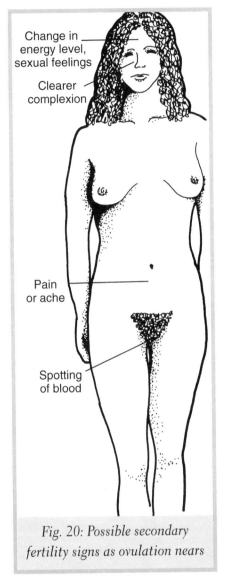

Fig. 20: *Possible secondary fertility signs as ovulation nears*

decrease in sexual feelings. Research has shown about 50 percent of women feel more sexual during menstruation, while about 50 percent experience this change around ovulation. Other women do not notice any change in sexual feelings throughout their cycle and this is normal for them.

Some women experience all of the secondary fertility signs described above, while others experience only a few. Sometimes signs are experienced during one cycle, but not the next. It is important not to confuse secondary fertility signs with premenstrual symptoms. Secondary fertility signs are experienced as ovulation approaches and/or during ovulation, while premenstrual symptoms are experienced anywhere from shortly after ovulation has occurred up to the time menstruation begins. These symptoms are quite different from secondary fertility signs and are often referred to as **premenstrual syndrome** (PMS). There are over 100 PMS symptoms, which can range from mild to severe, lasting as little as one day or as long as two weeks. PMS may or may not negatively effect a woman's life. Because these symptoms bother all too many women, tend to become worse as time goes by, and usually don't go away on their own, we have included some information about PMS.

Signs and Symptoms of PMS

As menstruation nears, the body's oil-producing glands secrete more oil, causing oilier skin and sometimes acne. Cramping, leg aches, and backaches can occur. A woman's body may hold more fluid, causing breast tenderness or pain. Itching of the nipples, headaches, fatigue, and mood changes can also occur. Some women notice a decrease in sexual feelings at this time.

The symptoms just mentioned are only a few of over 100 premenstrual symptoms that have been identified. (Please see the Bibliography for books that discuss premenstrual symptoms in detail as well as various ways to treat them.)

There are different theories about the causes and treatments of premenstrual syndrome. The bottom line is that PMS seems to be caused by several factors, not just one, and therefore the treatment probably needs to involve several approaches. Some people feel that the use of progesterone is the answer, though the majority of progesterone research hasn't shown that to be the case. Other research has shown that specific nutritional programs combined with specific vitamins, minerals, and essential fatty acids, such as flax seed oil, can be helpful for some women. Exercise and stress-reduction techniques have been shown to help as well. There are also several herbal and homeopathic programs that may relieve PMS. If you find that you, or someone you know, is experiencing bothersome physical and/or emotional changes one to fourteen days before menstruation, you should know that help is available. You can read information about premenstrual syndrome and discuss it with your physician, as well as contact organizations that have been formed to help women with this problem.

A Word about the Major and Secondary Fertility Signs

Please remember the goal of observing fertility signs is not to determine the exact day of ovulation. They can't be used for this purpose. Instead, when observed carefully, they will accurately show you when you are and are not fertile. Their changes will indicate well in advance when the time of ovulation is approaching as well as when it has occurred. Therefore, you will see and feel the beginning of your fertile time early enough in the fertility cycle to prevent or achieve a pregnancy. You will also know when your fertile time has ended.

TO REVIEW

During the fertility cycle you can experience various fertility signs—three major and several secondary ones.

MAJOR SIGNS

+ Changes in cervical mucus and vaginal sensations
+ Changes in basal body temperature
+ Changes in the cervix

POSSIBLE SECONDARY SIGNS—AS OVULATION APPROACHES

+ Clearing of complexion
+ Decrease in oil production, both in skin and in hair
+ Water retention

❖ Aches or pain in lower body

❖ Increased sensitivity in skin and breasts

❖ Increased energy level

❖ Increased or decreased sexual feelings

It is important for you to keep a record of as many fertility signs as possible on your fertility awareness chart. By doing this, you will be able to gain a clear understanding of the fertile and infertile times of your cycle. It will also increase your awareness of what is normal and healthy for you.

A Last Word about Observing Fertility Signs

The first step in learning about your own fertility pattern is to observe it carefully. To accomplish this, we recommend that you use as many fertility signs as you are comfortable with to prevent pregnancy. You will be establishing a new habit, learning accurate information, and developing your fertility awareness. Because of this, it is important that you check your fertility signs every day until you feel you have learned to do this well and are comfortable with your fertility pattern.

You need only about ten minutes each day to observe and record cervical mucus and BBT changes accurately. As you gain experience, you will get better and better at making these observations, decreasing the time spent. In fact, please remember that once you are confident about the changes in your fertility signs and you know when ovulation has passed and the fertile phase has ended, you do not need to check your signs for the remainder of that cycle.

Checking your fertility signs can be compared to the daily habit of brushing your teeth. It can be done automatically and regularly, and it only takes a few minutes. You pick up the toothbrush, squeeze the tube of toothpaste, and brush your teeth—without thinking. Placing a thermometer under your tongue and/or looking at cervical mucus and other signs can also become part of your daily routine. Before long this becomes habit, and you do it without giving it a second thought.

7

Charting the Way to Awareness

The first step in learning about your fertility pattern is to observe your fertility signs. The next step is to record them on a fertility awareness chart. You will then have a visual story of each fertility cycle. We'll first describe the way in which you should record your mucus and vaginal sensations, next how to record BBT and cervical changes. Then we'll discuss recording secondary fertility signs and other important information. You can see a sample fertility awareness chart, with all the relevant information for one cycle filled in, in Figure 21 on page 69. A blank chart for you to copy and use is included on the last page of this book.

Recording Cervical Mucus Changes

The following six symbols are used for recording cervical mucus changes on the chart:

1. "✳" represents menstrual bleeding.

2. "**S**" represents spotting of blood.

3. "**D**" represents dry days. These are the days when mucus is not **present for the entire day** and the outside of the vagina feels dry.

4. "**M**" represents sticky, pasty, and crumbly mucus that may feel slightly moist but does not feel obviously wet. The outside of the vagina feels dry or sticky.

5. "Ⓜ" represents wet mucus. These are the days when wet-feeling mucus is present and the outside of the vagina feels

wet. The mucus can be creamy or slippery and stretchy. Sometimes a wet sensation will be noticed on the outside of the vagina, but the mucus is not yet visible. In this situation the day is still considered an (M) , a wet mucus day.

6. "(M)" represents the one day that is the last day of slippery, stretchy, and very wet-feeling mucus and wet vaginal sensations. It is often called the "peak day." However, we will refer to it as the **last wet day**, because the name "peak day" might make you think it is the day when the mucus is the wettest or most slippery and stretchy, or when the greatest amount of mucus is present. It is important to remember this is not necessarily the case. It is also important to remember that **the last wet day can only be identified the day after it has passed.** It is very important to be on the lookout for this last day, especially if you are using your fertility signs as a way of preventing a pregnancy. (The Last Wet Day Rule is explained in Chapter 9.)

In addition to using these symbols, it can also be helpful to write down mucus descriptions in the Notes column on the chart. These descriptions would include the color, amount, and quality of the mucus. Some women use their own abbreviations and symbols when recording mucus descriptions. For example a "W" might be used to record white colored mucus and a "Y" for yellow mucus. A "+" sign might be used for a small amount of mucus and one "+" added each day a significantly greater amount of mucus is noticed. Please use whatever works for you to help you keep track of your own unique changes.

Recording Basal Body Temperature (BBT)

Basal body temperature (BBT) should be recorded in the temperature columns on the fertility awareness chart as follows:

1. Circle the temperature on the chart that is the same as your temperature for the day.

Note: A blank fertility awareness chart is printed on the last page of this book. Enlarge it on any photocopy machine to 150% and it will fit on a standard 8½ x 11-inch (letter size) sheet of paper. Please make copies of this chart for your personal use for charting your fertility signs. The chart may also be downloaded in pdf format from www.hunterhouse.com

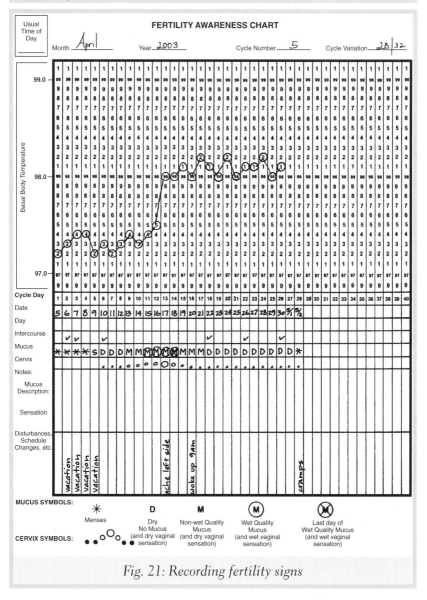

Fig. 21: Recording fertility signs

2. Connect each circle with a straight line—this makes the changes of the temperature clear to see.

3. The time you have chosen to take your temperature each day is written in the "usual time" space on the left-hand side of the chart.

4. If you awaken earlier or later than usual, are unable to take your BBT on a particular day, or experience anything else that you think might affect an accurate temperature reading, record this in the "Notes" column. When you can't take your BBT, you can place a question mark in the column for that day or just leave it blank.

Recording Cervical Changes

If you observe your cervical changes, you can record them in the following ways:

1. A small closed circle placed in the lower left-hand corner of the box [.] represents a low, closed cervix.

2. A larger circle [o] represents the cervix as its opening enlarges. Every day the opening feels larger, the circle becomes more open.

3. As the cervix becomes higher in the vaginal canal, the circles are placed higher in the boxes. [O]

4. S represents a soft cervix. [O s]

5. F represents a firm cervix. [. F]

   S and F are also recorded in the boxes.

Special note: When the fertility signs are not the same throughout the day, always record the fertility sign change that seems like the *most fertile sign* of the day. This is a conservative approach and one that will serve you well if you are using your fertility signs to prevent pregnancy. For example, if you do not see any mucus in the morning and your vaginal sensations are dry, but you notice a small amount of pasty mucus in the evening with dry vaginal sensations, the small amount of pasty mucus is recorded as the mucus of the day by using the letter **M**. This appearance of mucus is an indication that estrogen is just beginning to rise and therefore is the most fertile sign of the day.

If you feel wet, creamy mucus in the morning with wet vaginal sensations and pasty, sticky, non-wet mucus in the evening with a sticky vaginal sensation, it is still considered a wet day and is recorded with an Ⓜ . Wet mucus is a more fertile sign than pasty, sticky, non-wet mucus. If you feel the cervix in a low position in the morning and afternoon, but by evening it feels higher, the higher cervix observation ⬚ is recorded, as a higher cervix indicates a potentially more fertile time than a lower cervix does.

If you experience any change in your cervical mucus that makes you feel as though you have a vaginal infection, if you have semen, spermicide or vaginal medication in the vaginal area, or if you are unable to check your mucus on a particular day for whatever reason, place a question mark on your chart on that particular cycle day or days. It is also helpful to write a description of what you are seeing and feeling if the discharge appears abnormal for you. If the symptoms don't go away within a day or so, or are very uncomfortable, please be examined by your clinician. Always make a note of the reason for your being unable to accurately check your mucus on a particular day, such as "vaginal medication."

Recording Secondary Fertility Signs

Secondary fertility signs are recorded as follows:

1. All physical and/or emotional changes experienced during each fertility cycle are recorded in the "Notes" column.

2. These changes should be recorded on the exact day that they are experienced.

   Everything and anything you feel or observe should be written down to help you learn about your own special fertility cycle.

The more information you record, the less you will need to remember, and the greater will be the rewards and discoveries you experience as your body undergoes its changes during the fertility cycle.

The key to all of the information in this book is that your body talks to you! It's letting you know what is occurring in your fertility cycle—a pattern of events and changes that will provide a silent but powerful personal language, the language of fertility.

Completing the Fertility Chart: An Example

Figure 21 on page 67 is an example of how to complete the fertility awareness chart.

- ✦ The usual time of day the temperature is taken, and the month and year of the cycle being recorded, should all be noted. In this case, the usual time of temperature taking is 8:00 A.M., and the month and year of the cycle are April, 2003.

- ✦ The cycle number should be filled in with the number of the cycle being observed. The first cycle you chart will be labeled number one, the second will be number two, and so on. In this example the chart records cycle number five.

- ✦ Cycle variation represents the number of days in the shortest and longest cycle. In this chart, the number of days in the shortest fertility cycle was 28 and the number of days in the longest fertility cycle was 32, hence the 28/32 notation at the top right of the chart. The cycle variation notation should always reflect **the lengths of up to the six most recent fertility cycles**. If a woman does not know the lengths of her six most recent fertility cycles, or if she has just discontinued taking birth control pills, had a baby, or experienced any situation that stopped ovulation for one or more months, she will record her cycle lengths as she experiences them with each cycle of charting her fertility signs.

❖ The length of the previous fertility cycle should be recorded as well.

❖ The fertility signs the woman chooses to observe are recorded on a daily basis along with any other descriptions of mucus, vaginal sensations, and secondary fertility signs.

❖ Any changes in lifestyle should be noted in the appropriate columns at the bottom of the chart. On our sample chart, on cycle days two to five, a vacation is noted. Although a vacation may not change the fertility cycle, it is noted just in case it does.

To review this chart:

❖ The woman had knowledge of her previous four fertility cycles, and this was the fifth cycle she was charting. Thus she has filled in "5" as the cycle number.

❖ The shortest cycle of her previous four cycles was 28 days; the longest cycle was 32 days. Therefore, her cycle variation up to this point is 28/32. When she completes her next chart, she will have a full record of the lengths of six cycles.

❖ Since this cycle was 27 days long, her cycle variation on her next chart would be noted 27/32.

❖ She usually takes her temperature at 8:00 A.M. This is marked in the "usual time" space.

❖ In the "Notes" column, she recorded pain on her left side on day 13 of her fertility cycle. On day 28 she experienced menstrual cramps, which she also noted. She recorded the fact that she awoke later than usual on cycle day 16. She also recorded the days she had intercourse by placing a " ✔ " in the column marked "intercourse."

Please note that the more complete a chart is, the more accurate a method of family planning you will create for yourself.

8

Using Fertility Awareness Information to Become Pregnant

How would you answer the question, "Can a women become pregnant at any time?" With the information you have learned up to this point, you would respond with something like, "No, a woman can only become pregnant if she has intercourse during her fertile days." If a woman wants to become pregnant, she must know how to identify her fertile days. With this knowledge, she can be sure to have intercourse at some point during these days in order to achieve a pregnancy. Unfortunately, all too many women do not know this and experience difficulty becoming pregnant simply because of a lack of knowledge about their own fertility cycle.

Instructions for Planning a Pregnancy

Perhaps you have been trying to become pregnant for a while or want to become pregnant ASAP! Or you may be thinking about pregnancy, yet aren't quite ready to become pregnant at this time. In any of these situations, we would like to suggest you take the time to observe your fertility signs (at least cervical mucus and basal body temperature) for a month or more before you try to achieve a pregnancy. We know this is easy to ask and we also know that it is not always easy to do. When some women have been trying to become pregnant or are ready to begin trying, waiting one or two more cycles to learn their fertility signs is not a welcome thought! However, please consider this fact: If you give your-self time to learn about your mucus and BBT changes, you will then be able to identify accurately when your fertile days begin during future fer-tility cycles. In addition, if you learn about your fertility patterns before pregnancy, you can develop the understanding necessary to use your fer-tility signs to avoid pregnancy after the baby is born, should you chose to do so. And finally, if you notice an unusual fertility sign pattern for a couple of cycles, you will know to discuss this with your clinician. You may learn of a problem that can be diagnosed early, and therefore treated early, so that you can become pregnant. As you can see, taking the time to learn about your fertility signs has many benefits.

If you do choose to give yourself the time to observe your signs for a cycle or two and plan to have intercourse, please consider using a male condom, preferably one that is NOT treated with a lubricant or spermi-cide. When semen mixes with cervical mucus, it makes learning about mucus changes difficult. Used properly, a condom will prevent semen from mixing with the mucus. If this choice is not workable for you, per-haps you and your partner would feel comfortable experiencing other forms of lovemaking besides intercourse. By doing this, again, you won't be introducing semen into the vagina. This will allow you to observe your mucus accurately.

Once you have observed your fertility signs for at least one fertility cycle, and you are comfortable identifying the beginning of your fertile time, you are ready to try to become pregnant! If you are using mucus changes to identify the beginning of the fertile time, the ideal approach is to abstain or use a condom after your period ends so that you are able to determine the first day you begin to experience either wet vaginal sensations and/or wet mucus. Since this is your body's signal you are ap-proaching ovulation, *you should try to begin having intercourse on that day.* Continue having intercourse as often as you like after the wet mucus begins and until the day after your basal body temperature rises. If your partner's semen has a normal amount of sperm in it, research has shown that having intercourse a few days in a row shouldn't decrease your chances of becoming pregnant.

Having intercourse the day before or on the day of the rise in your basal body temperature will probably give you the greatest possibility of pregnancy. However, since you cannot predict when your temperature will rise, *the wet cervical mucus is the best indicator of the beginning of the fertile time*. If you are observing your cervical changes, a high, soft, and open cervix is another indication of your most fertile days.

Once your temperature rises, you should continue taking it for the remainder of the cycle if you want to use it as a form of pregnancy test. If your basal body temperature remains high longer than 20 days, and you don't experience your usual menstrual bleeding, it can mean that you are pregnant. If this occurs, it is important that you have a pregnancy test and be examined so that the pregnancy can be confirmed and the date the baby will be born can be determined. Another reason for this examination is the need to begin early obstetrical care so that your pregnancy is as healthy as it can be.

TO REVIEW

✤ Observe your fertility signs for one cycle or more. If you want to learn about the mucus pattern, abstinence from intercourse or use of a non-lubricated condom during these cycles will enable accurate observation of the mucus changes.

✤ Once you've decided to become pregnant, abstain or use a condom after your menstrual bleeding ends. When your fertile time begins, it's time to put away the condoms. In order to achieve pregnancy, intercourse must take place when you experience wet, fertile mucus.

✤ Continue taking your basal body temperature after the rise. A BBT that remains elevated beyond the usual cycle length is an excellent sign that pregnancy has been achieved.

Becoming Pregnant

Again, please remember if a man has no reason to suspect that he has a fertility problem, or if his semen analysis is normal, having intercourse every day during the fertile time does not seem to decrease a couple's chance for pregnancy. However, some men have a low sperm count or a problem related to the sperm movement. In this situation it is advisable for the couple to have intercourse every other day during the fertile time. This maximizes the number of sperm in the semen.

Intercourse must occur during wet mucus days to achieve pregnancy, but it doesn't mean intercourse shouldn't take place during other days in the cycle. Some couples who are trying to become pregnant change their usual sexual lifestyle in a way that isn't pleasing to them. Instead of enjoying each other sexually whenever they desire, they abstain from intercourse and from other ways of being affectionate during infertile times of the fertility cycle.

There is no reason why intercourse can't take place at any time early in the fertility cycle. However, since you want to be able to detect the first day of wet mucus and a wet vaginal sensation, you can use condoms. Another option is to abstain the day after you have had intercourse to allow adequate time for semen to flow out of the vagina. The day after the abstinence day would then be a mucus checking day. If you experience wet mucus, you will know your fertile time has begun. For example, let's say you see some sticky, pasty mucus and the vaginal area feels dry on Monday. Since you didn't see or feel any wet mucus, you decide to have intercourse on that day. You feel wetness in the vaginal area the next morning on Tuesday because you had intercourse. You decide to abstain on Tuesday to allow enough time for the semen to leave the vaginal area. You then check your mucus on Wednesday. You notice some sticky mucus in the morning, but by the afternoon and night time, the mucus definitely feels wet. You now know your fertile time has started and its time to try to become pregnant.

Perhaps you don't want to check your cervical mucus to determine the beginning of your fertile days. If so, there is another option available to you, one that works well for some women who are trying to become pregnant. Subtract 19 from the length of your previous fertility cycle to determine what will most likely be the first day of your fertile phase of the next cycle. For example, if the cycle you just finished was 30 days long, subtract 19 and you will know that your fertile phase will probably begin on day 11 of the next cycle.

This is called the 19 Day Rule and should NOT be used for pregnancy prevention, only as an aid in becoming pregnant. It is a technique that can be used if your cycle lengths are fairly regular—for example, if your cycle lengths don't vary in length beyond two to four days. If your cycles vary in length for a greater number of days, or if they are truly irregular, this option will probably not be useful for you. In these situations, cervical mucus is much more helpful.

A Few Pregnancy Preparation Issues

In addition to learning fertility signs and the proper timing for intercourse, the couple desiring a pregnancy should consider a few other issues.

First, it is advisable to have a complete medical checkup before becoming pregnant. This examination gives you and your doctor an opportunity to discuss any medical problems that might exist. For example, if you are taking medications, it is important to know whether they will be harmful if taken during pregnancy. An examination will also provide the opportunity, if necessary, for certain tests to be performed, such as for rubella (German measles), sickle cell anemia, and Tay-Sachs disease.

Another issue is selection of the child's sex through special methods of timing intercourse. Several sources have indicated that pregnancy occurring as a result of intercourse a few days before the thermal shift (in other words, when wet mucus first appears) increases the possibility of the baby being a girl. Intercourse occurring near the day of the thermal shift and/or day of the most abundant wet, slippery mucus increases the possibility of a boy.

Although studies have been conducted and books have been written on this subject, planning the child's sex seems to have been successful for only a small percentage of couples. It seems as though, regardless of what method or technique a couple uses to attempt to have a baby boy or girl, the end result is still about a 50 percent chance of having a girl and a 50 percent chance of having a boy. This is approximately the odds when a couple is not using any method at all for sex selection. There are, however, special ways of preparing sperm in a laboratory that will increase the chances of having a baby boy. If this is something you wish to pursue, you can contact a fertility specialist in your area. Either the specialist will offer the specific technique for sex selection or will be able to refer you to a physician who does offer it.

Infertility

Approximately 15 percent of all couples have some difficulty achieving a pregnancy. Unfortunately, many of them don't know when to seek medical attention, and they are unaware of the facts about infertility tests and treatments. Other couples delay seeking medical attention because of fear. They are fearful of having a problem that cannot be corrected. Some are not aware that there are successful treatments for some of the causes of infertility.

On the average, it takes a couple three to four months to achieve a pregnancy. About 85 percent of couples attempting to achieve a pregnancy will succeed after one year of trying. There are many reasons why the other 15 percent do not succeed. Some causes are related to fertility problems with the man, others to fertility problems with the woman. Sometimes, both partners will have problems. If a couple has not achieved a pregnancy after having intercourse two or more times during the fertile days for six to nine fertility cycles, we advise a consultation with a fertility specialist. It usually takes some time to undergo fertility testing to attempt to identify the cause of the problem. If treatment is available, it usually takes time for it to be successful. Therefore, waiting longer than six to nine months is probably not the best decision to make. When consulting a physician, please consider choosing a physician who specializes in fertility problems. All too often, when a couple is having difficulty and seeks care through someone not very knowledgeable about fertility, they don't receive the help they need to become pregnant.

Infertility and the Man

The most common fertility problems in men are related to either a low number of sperm in the semen or poor activity (movement) of the sperm. The causes of these problems include:

* ❖ infection in any part of the man's reproductive system
* ❖ exposure to chemicals
* ❖ medical illnesses
* ❖ prescription and nonprescription drugs
* ❖ dilated veins in the scrotum (varicocele)
* ❖ excessive intake of alcohol, caffeine, or recreational drugs
* ❖ poor nutrition
* ❖ smoking
* ❖ stress

Other causes of infertility are abnormalities of the testes and the passageways necessary for the normal travel of sperm and seminal fluid. These abnormalities can be due to improperly developed parts of the re-productive system, infection, or operations on or near the reproductive organs.

The first test used to check the number and quality of sperm is called *semen analysis*. If the test result is not normal, additional special tests and procedures are performed to identify the cause and possible treatment of the problem. A man's semen is often tested to determine if he is allergic to his own sperm and if the sperm are able to fertilize an egg.

Infertility and the Woman

ANOVULATION—no ovulation or infrequent ovulation—is a common cause of infertility in women, and is often successfully treated by the use of fertility drugs. Two of the more common reasons for anovulation are:

* ❖ disturbances in the usual ways the hormones are supposed to work that cannot be explained (unfortunately, often ovulation doesn't happen and the cause can't be determined)

❖ physical and emotional stress (discussed in Chapter 10)

❖ poor nutrition, eating disorders

❖ excessive intake of alcohol or recreational drugs

Allergy to the man's sperm is also a cause of infertility. Another cause is cervical problems: Cervical infections or surgery performed on the cervix can lead to

❖ inadequate production of cervical mucus

❖ production of cervical mucus that may not be of the quality necessary to allow sperm to live and pass through it to reach the egg

Cervical mucus can also contain substances that inactivate the sperm, in the same manner that the body produces antibodies that inactivate bacteria and viruses when it is fighting off an infection or illness. A common treatment for this problem is antibiotic therapy to clear up infections.

Problems of the uterus and fallopian tubes can also cause infertility. An infection occurring in and around the internal reproductive organs (pelvic infection) can cause scarring of the fallopian tubes. This scarring may prevent the sperm from reaching the egg or the egg from entering the tube. Sometimes this can be corrected by tubal surgery.

ENDOMETRIOSIS (en-do-me-tree-o-sis) is a cause of infertility that can occur at any age but seems to be experienced more often by older women who have delayed having children. It is believed that endometriosis develops when the tissue that normally lines the inside of the uterus flows up through the fallopian tubes into the area of the ovaries. The presence of this tissue can cause scarring that may prevent the sperm from reaching the egg or the egg from entering the tube. Endometriosis is often treated by surgery to remove the tissue and scarring. Hormone therapy is another treatment used to reduce growth of the endometrial tissue.

Other Causes of Infertility

The cause of the infertility problem is unknown in about 5 percent of all couples who have an infertility evaluation. Some of these couples will achieve a pregnancy at some time without treatment of any kind. For others who have particularly stressful life situations, pregnancy may occur after they have dealt successfully with their stress. Some are able to do this by themselves, while others may need to seek the assistance of a professional skilled in helping people with this problem—a psychologist, counselor, or psychiatrist.

Improper Timing of Intercourse

It may take a long time for a couple to achieve a pregnancy simply because they are not having intercourse on their fertile days. Observing fertility signs can often enable a couple to achieve a pregnancy sooner because they have intercourse when the woman is fertile.

A Word about Fertility Problems, Tests, and Treatments

The information we have provided here is an extremely basic overview of fertility problems. Tests and treatments are changing every day, thanks to technological advances and an increase in research efforts in the field of fertility. If you feel you need to learn more about these areas, we encourage you to talk with a fertility expert or, at a minimum, read one or more books on fertility. You will find some suggested titles in the Bibliography. Make sure the books you choose are written by physicians who are experts in fertility! Many books that are not written by fertility specialists include inaccurate or outdated information, or an interpretation of information that has not been studied well. These will not help you and may only cause you unnecessary confusion and fear, or perhaps even delay you from receiving the correct treatment.

Feelings and Infertility

Infertility is usually an extremely difficult life situation for a couple. Since many women and men have a strong desire for a child, the couple unable to have a child of their own may experience feelings of anger and frustration, as well as guilt, depression, and sadness. These feelings can be devastating to the couple and their relationship. Because of this, it can be helpful to talk with someone who can provide support and understanding. An infertility organization, therapist, counselor, or spiritual guide can provide this support and be beneficial to couples working through this very difficult time.

We mentioned a few reasons why we have chosen not to discuss all of the many tests, causes, and treatments of fertility problems. This is not because we don't feel the subject of infertility is important—quite the opposite. A thorough discussion of fertility and infertility problems deserves its own book, of which there are many. Examples of several books about fertility are included in the Bibliography, and the website www.ihr.com is also a good source for infertility resources.

There is also an organization of men and women, Resolve, committed to helping people with infertility problems. It is based in Boston and has chapters in many major cities. For more information, contact Resolve, PO Box 474, Belmont MA 02178 (617-623-0744).

Scientific Advances to Help Couples Achieve Pregnancy

There are various products available to the public that can be used to closely predict the day of ovulation. Available in many drugstores, these ovulation predictor kits are based on the fact that the amount of a hormone made by the pituitary gland, called **luteinizing hormone** (LH), increases greatly approximately 24–36 hours before ovulation.

When a woman collects a sample of her urine on specific days during each fertility cycle, and mixes the urine with a chemical included in the kits, the urine will change color. This color change indicates that a sudden increase in LH has occurred and that ovulation will usually begin within 24–36 hours.

Some women choose to use an ovulation predictor test to help confirm that ovulation is taking place as well as to determine when intercourse is most likely to result in pregnancy.

At the present time, it is unknown whether the chances of achieving a pregnancy are greater for women who use these tests as compared to women who time intercourse when indicated by the presence of fertile mucus.

If a woman, regardless of whether or not she is trying to prevent or achieve a pregnancy, is unsure whether she is ovulating, the information from using one of these tests and keeping track of BBT and cervical mucus may give her the information she needs to confirm ovulation. However, it is advisable to seek the advice of a physician in these cases. No test is 100 percent accurate: If a woman does not think she is ovulating, it is important to find out whether this is definitely the case, and if so, the reason for it. Other tests for determining the approach of ovulation are available, such as tests that measure changes in the saliva of the mouth or certain chemical changes in the vagina that reflect rising levels of estrogen, and therefore a time of fertility. Research regarding the effectiveness of these tests in helping couples conceive is limited. This doesn't mean they are not helpful. They can help some women conceive without using fertility signs. However, at this point, we recommend that, if you use them, you do so in combination with observing mucus and BBT.

There are also computer programs that help couples identify their fertile time. They may or may not be more effective than observing one's fertility signs. It depends on the technology and data being used. Again, no studies have been done comparing groups of couples who observed their fertility signs and had intercourse during the fertile time versus those who used a microcomputer or software program to identify the fertile days. In addition, if a woman does not ovulate regularly, these may not be useful at all. The decision to use forms of technology to help conceive is a personal one, given that they may or may not offer any advantage beyond what basic fertility sign observation and recording offers.

9

The Natural Family Planning Method

You've learned about fertility signs, the ways in which they change throughout a fertility cycle, and how they are observed and recorded. Now let's look at the instructions you will need to follow to determine when your fertile and infertile days begin and end. These instructions are called natural family planning rules, and there are several available for your use. Some are very conservative, resulting in the highest effectiveness possible. These usually require more days of abstinence than other, slightly less effective rules.

Other rules are somewhat less conservative and their effectiveness rate is a little bit lower; however, it is important to know that the less conservative approach still offers a great, effective method of family planning. The rules you choose to follow will depend upon the fertility sign(s) you decide to observe and how conservative a method of NFP you want to use.

Please remember one very important fact: No matter what rules you decide to use, a woman does not have to have intercourse to get pregnant! This was discussed in the section on male fertility and is critical information that many women and men do not know. As strange as it may sound, pregnancy can happen if semen comes into contact with the vaginal opening during a woman's fertile days. The reason for this is that when fertile mucus is being produced, it flows down the vagina and to the vaginal opening. If sperm come into contact with the mucus, the sperm can swim up the vagina, through the cervix, and eventually down the fallopian tube where they may meet with an egg! The best way to avoid this from happening is to prevent sperm from getting anywhere near the vaginal opening. For example, a man should not ejaculate close to the outside of the vaginal opening.

The natural family planning rules are used to determine:

* The **infertile phase before ovulation**, during which time you can have intercourse with little chance of pregnancy.

* When the **fertile phase** begins. This phase lasts several days. It starts a few days before ovulation, continues during ovulation, and ends a few days after ovulation. If intercourse takes place during this phase, the chance of pregnancy is great.

* The end of the fertile phase and the beginning of the **infertile phase after ovulation**. The infertile phase begins a few days after ovulation, lasts several days, and ends when a new cycle begins.

During the infertile phase after ovulation, intercourse may occur with a **very unlikely** chance of pregnancy. In fact, when the rules are used and followed carefully, there is almost no chance of pregnancy during this phase.

NFP Rules Used to Determine the Infertile Phase Before Ovulation: The Most Conservative Rules

Menstrual Abstinence Rule

ABSTAIN DURING MENSTRUAL BLEEDING.

Surprised? If you're like many people, you learned that it wasn't possible for a woman to become pregnant from having intercourse during menstruation. However, this is not always the case; although the possibility is small, (perhaps only 1–5 percent), it still exists. And the first reason for this is early ovulation. A woman can ovulate soon after her menstrual period ends. Some women experience this every fertility cycle because these women usually have normal cycles which are less than 25 days long.

As you recall, ovulation usually takes place 12 to 16 days before menstruation starts. Using a 24-day cycle as an example, let's subtract 12 from 24 ($24 - 12 = 12$) and 16 from 24 ($24 - 16 = 8$). A woman who has a 24-day-long cycle would ovulate between cycle days 8 and 12. The earliest she would probably ovulate is the 8th day of her cycle.

On the other hand, if we take a cycle length of 28 days, the earliest ovulation would probably occur is cycle day 12: $28 - 16 = 12$ and $28 - 12 = 16$. A woman who has 28-day cycles usually ovulates between cycle days 12 and 16. Fortunately, most women don't ovulate close to the end of their periods because they normally have cycles that are longer than 25 days.

If most women have cycles that are usually longer than 25 days, can they ever ovulate earlier than usual? The answer is yes! Earlier-than-usual ovulation can be a result of any number of factors, including illness, stress, a change in lifestyle (e.g., exercise or nutritional habits), or for reasons not yet understood. It can be a part of the normal aging process. An earlier-than-usual ovulation is not necessarily considered abnormal, but merely one way in which a woman's body is reacting to a change in her life. However, it can be problematic if a woman does not want to become pregnant.

Unfortunately, no one can predict in advance when ovulation will happen. Imagine the woman who usually has 30-day cycles. If you subtract 12 from 30 ($30 - 12 = 18$) and 16 from 30 ($30 - 16 = 14$), you know that she usually ovulates between cycle days 14 and 18. However, let's say she gets her period, and because she recently began a new exercise program, the timing of her ovulation has temporarily been changed. This time she is going to ovulate on cycle day 8. Does she know this is going to happen? No! When a woman is menstruating, she has no idea whether she might ovulate early. Let's say by the fifth day of her period, her cervix is producing great fertile mucus that she can't see because of the presence of blood. She has intercourse on day 5, sperm live until cycle day 8 when she ovulates, the sperm and egg meet, and she becomes pregnant. Again, this does not happen very often, but it is possible. Now let's say this same woman who usually has 30-day cycles and who therefore usually ovulates between cycle days 14 and 18 is going to ovulate on day 10. Her period ends and she begins to watch for mucus and pays attention to her vaginal sensations. During the cycle in which she is going to ovulate earlier, she notices cervical mucus on cycle day 6, right after her period ends. Because she has learned NFP well, she knows her body is signaling her that she is probably going to ovulate earlier than usual and therefore knows her fertile phase is beginning earlier. That being the case, she begins to abstain on cycle day 6 and continues to abstain until she knows her fertile time has ended.

The example we've just given makes sense because, as you have learned, cervical mucus begins to be produced several days before ovulation. With an early ovulation, a woman will probably observe the same changes in her mucus and vaginal sensations she always has but she will see and feel them earlier in her cycle.

Another example: Joanne usually has fertility cycles that are at least 27 days long. She usually sees cervical mucus appear around day 10, and it becomes very wet by day 14.

However, one cycle she noticed cervical mucus five days before she was used to seeing it. It appeared on cycle day 6, one day after her menstrual period ended (Figure 22). She remembered that mucus appearing earlier than usual was probably an indication she was going to ovulate early, and so she knew her fertile phase had begun earlier. Because she did not want to become pregnant, she abstained from intercourse and continued to observe her mucus as usual until she was sure her fertile phase had ended.

Abstinence during bleeding is also recommended as a very conservative measure because a woman may assume she is experiencing men-

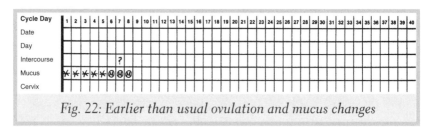

Fig. 22: Earlier than usual ovulation and mucus changes

strual bleeding when she is actually bleeding for some other reason. She may actually be ovulating! Occasionally a woman can bleed with ovulation even if she had never experienced this during previous cycles. Sometimes a woman can experience bleeding due to a hormonal imbalance or for some other reason and coincidentally ovulate during the bleeding or within a day or so after the bleeding ends. Non-menstrual bleeding can be heavier or lighter than a woman's normal menstrual flow and may not last as long as her usual period. It also often appears at a different time of the cycle. Yet, as you can imagine, a woman might begin to bleed and think "I'm getting my period earlier than usual. It's okay to have intercourse." If a woman assumes this is a normal menstrual period and has intercourse, and fertile mucus is present, again, she won't be able to see or feel it. If she ovulates, and sperm are waiting for the egg, pregnancy can result.

The two examples we've just given are not common—in fact, they are quite rare. Yet anyone who wants the most conservative method of natural family planning will probably choose to abstain from intercourse during bleeding.

Some women don't object to this rule because they don't enjoy intercourse during menstrual bleeding or find it objectionable for religious or other personal reasons. However, other women don't like this rule since intercourse during menstrual bleeding is pleasurable for them. Some women even find they have an increase in sexual feelings during menstruation. If you want to have intercourse during bleeding, you will learn later in this chapter how to determine if the bleeding you are experiencing is truly menstrual bleeding and when you can very safely have intercourse during this time with a minimal chance of pregnancy.

Dry Day Rule

INTERCOURSE CAN OCCUR DURING THE NIGHT OF ANY DRY DAY.

Can intercourse begin the day after menstrual bleeding ends? Yes, if a dry day is experienced. Many women experience one or more dry days

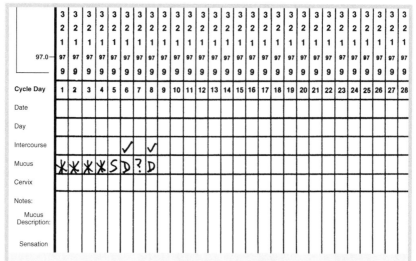

Fig. 23: The Dry Day Rule

Heidi experienced a dry day on cycle day 6. Intercourse took place on that night and a wet discharge was experienced on cycle day 7. This was recorded as a question mark "?" because there was no way of determining whether this discharge was mucus, semen, or a combination of both. Therefore, abstinence was followed on cycle day 7. Since cycle day 8 was a dry day, this couple decided to have intercourse that night.

It is important to note that not all women experience a wet discharge the day after intercourse. Some women have stated that if they urinate and bathe after intercourse, they don't see or feel semen in the vaginal area the next day. If this is the case and you are sure you are experiencing a completely dry day on the day following intercourse, you can have intercourse again during that night.

after menses. As previously discussed, dry days are ones in which no mucus is seen and vaginal sensations are dry throughout the day and into the evening. The fact that no mucus is seen means that ovulation is probably not going to occur for at least a few days, and possibly not until several days later. In addition, without the right kind of mucus, sperm cannot live and travel in the reproductive system. Therefore, the possibility of pregnancy is extremely low—in fact, almost zero—if intercourse occurs during a dry day.

The Dry Day Rule specifically states that intercourse can only occur during the *night* of a dry day. Waiting to have intercourse until the nighttime allows you to watch for mucus and wet vaginal sensations throughout the day. It gives you ample time to make sure that no mucus is on its way down to the vaginal opening. Remember, you may not see or feel mucus in the morning and afternoon, but as you walk around during the day, if mucus is being produced, gravity will help it travel down to the vaginal opening where you will see it later in the day.

Let's assume you use the Dry Day Rule and have intercourse tonight because it was a dry day for you. You did not see any mucus and your vaginal sensations were dry every time you checked throughout the day and evening. You have intercourse and tomorrow you experience a wet **vaginal discharge.** You need to ask yourself: "Is this discharge semen? Is it mucus? Is it a combination of both?" If the wet discharge is mucus and you have intercourse again, you could become pregnant. It can be very difficult if not impossible to tell the difference between semen and cervical mucus. Therefore, you should take the following steps to determine whether the discharge was semen or mucus: Abstain from intercourse for 24 hours. If the wet discharge was semen, it will pass out of the vaginal opening and be gone within 24 hours. Once the 24 hours have passed, check for mucus and a change in vaginal sensations. If you have another dry day, intercourse can again take place during that night.

TIPS FOR GETTING RID OF SEMEN Some women find that they can eliminate the semen in their vaginas by urinating after intercourse, performing Kegel exercises, and washing the semen from the vaginal area. Therefore, when they awaken the next day, they do not have a wet vaginal discharge. The semen is gone. They check mucus and their vaginal sensations throughout the day and find it is a dry day. Because they are not experiencing anything that indicates a possible fertile day, they can have intercourse again during that night.

NFP Rule Used to Determine the Beginning of the Fertile Phase

Early Mucus Rule

ABSTINENCE BEGINS (AND THE FERTILE PHASE STARTS) WHEN ANY MUCUS IS SEEN AND/OR WET VAGINAL SENSATIONS ARE EXPERIENCED, WHICHEVER COMES FIRST.

You know that at some point before ovulation, cervical mucus will begin to be produced. When this begins depends on the woman's cycle length and her own unique fertility pattern. It can also begin on different days during different fertility cycles. For example, a woman's fertile phase might begin on day 10 of one cycle and on day 12 of another cycle.

As we have previously discussed:

1. Some women can experience mucus on the day after menstrual bleeding ends.

2. Other women have dry days first, then begin to see mucus.

3. Usually the first type of mucus seen is pasty and sticky, and does not feel wet. This is a typical infertile type of mucus and it might seem as if intercourse should be able to take place when it is present. However, as you know, it may take up to a day for mucus to travel from inside the cervix to the outside of the vagina. Because of this, if infertile-type mucus is seen at the vaginal opening, is it possible there could be some wet, fertile mucus way up in the cervix that has not yet traveled down to the vaginal opening? Yes, this is possible, and there is no way for anyone to be absolutely positive that is not the case. Some suggest a woman squeeze her cervix with two fingers and try to force mucus out of the cervix and see if it is the wet, fertile kind. There is no research on this technique, and we don't recommend depending on it to prevent pregnancy. In addition, doing this could irritate the cervix. Therefore, to be most conservative, the fertile phase begins when *any type* of mucus

appears, even when the vaginal sensations are dry. The mucus could be non-wet or sticky. It doesn't matter.

4. If wet vaginal sensations are experienced, the fertile phase has begun. This is the case even when no mucus or non-wet mucus is observed. As strange as it may sound, sometimes, a woman can experience wet vaginal sensations even when she is unable to see any wet mucus. Since this could be a signal that wet mucus is going to begin to travel down to the vaginal opening, wet vaginal sensations should be considered a signal that the fertile phase has started.

NFP Rules Used to Determine the Infertile Days Before Ovulation: Less Conservative Rules

The *most* conservative NFP rules to use before ovulation are

1. Abstinence should be followed during menstrual bleeding.

2. Intercourse can take place on the night of any dry day.

There are two more rules that you can use to know when you can and cannot have intercourse before the fertile phase begins. These are the **Menses Rule** and the **21 Day Rule**. Both are very effective rules (about 95–99 percent effective) and can increase the number of days available for intercourse.

Menses Rule

INTERCOURSE CAN OCCUR DURING THE FIRST FIVE DAYS OF THE FERTILITY CYCLE AS LONG AS THE MOST RECENT SIX CYCLES WERE LONGER THAN 25 DAYS AND OVULATION OCCURRED DURING THE PREVIOUS FERTILITY CYCLE.

Research has shown that when a woman's usual cycle length is longer than 25 days, the possibility of an earlier-than-usual ovulation is very small. Research has also shown that, even if a woman ovulates earlier than usual, the possibility of pregnancy is very low when intercourse occurs during the first five days of the fertility cycle—as long as the woman ovulated during the previous cycle. The most accurate way for a woman to know whether she has ovulated is by observing a rise in her BBT about 12 to 16 days before menstrual bleeding started. The BBT should rise to at least 0.3°F or 0.05°C higher than it has been and stay high for several days. If the woman knows she ovulated, she will also know that the bleeding she experiences about 12 to 16 days later is menstrual bleeding and not bleeding with ovulation or bleeding for some other reason.

In addition, if the woman's cycles are usually longer than 25 days, she knows she does not usually ovulate close to the end of her menstrual period. This means the chances of pregnancy are extremely low if intercourse takes place during the first five days of her cycle.

Remember: The first five days of the fertility cycle are safe for intercourse. This means that if a woman's menstrual bleeding lasts for three days, every day of bleeding plus two days after her period ends are safe for intercourse. If bleeding lasts for six days, only the first five days of bleeding are safe for intercourse. For those women who are comfortable having intercourse during their menstrual bleeding, this rule provides days early in the cycle when the possibility of pregnancy is extremely low.

After menstrual bleeding ends, the Dry Day Rule can be used. This rule is an excellent one for those women who wish to observe their mucus. By using this rule, women can know when to have intercourse safely before the fertile phase begins. However, some women ask, "Is there another way I can know when my fertile time is going to begin, whether or not I am observing mucus?" There is a way! Women who do not want to observe mucus, or who want to know in advance when their fertile phase is probably going to begin, can use the 21 Day Rule. This rule is actually a simple mathematical formula that provides a woman with the length of the infertile time before ovulation.

21 Day Rule

THE NUMBER OF DAYS IN THE INFERTILE PHASE BEFORE OVULATION IS DETERMINED BY SUBTRACTING 21 FROM THE TOTAL NUMBER OF DAYS IN THE SHORTEST OF THE SIX MOST RECENT FERTILITY CYCLES.

This interesting rule is extremely effective because it is based on the following:

1. Ovulation will take place about 12 to 16 days before menstrual bleeding begins.

2. Sperm are able to survive and fertilize an egg for up to 5 days when fertile mucus is present. $16 + 5 = 21$

3. The number of days in the shortest cycle experienced during the six most recent, consecutive cycles minus 21 equals the length of the infertile phase before ovulation. The infertile phase before ovulation always starts on the first day of the menstrual period.

If you want to use this rule, subtract 21 from the length of the shortest fertility cycle that you have had in the last six cycles. You do not need to have charted fertility signs for these six cycles; you need to know only their length to use this rule. By subtracting 21 from the number of days in your shortest cycle, you will know the number of infertile days you have beginning on the first day of menstruation.

EXAMPLE: Susan marks on her calendar when she began menstruating for the last six cycles. She finds that her cycles varied from 29–32 days in length. Therefore, the shortest cycle was 29 days long. Susan subtracts 21 from 29, to get 8 ($29 - 21 = 8$). Therefore, Susan's infertile phase before ovulation is 8 days long. She can have intercourse from the first day of her fertility cycle up to and including day 8 of her cycle whenever she wants, with a minimal chance of pregnancy. Her fertile phase begins on the day after her infertile phase ends according to the 21 Day Rule. In this case, the fertile phase starts on cycle day 9.

EXAMPLE: Ann's fertility cycles during the months of December through May (six cycles) were 28–30 days long. If she subtracts 21 from the shortest of these cycles (28 days), she has an infertile phase of 7 days (28 – 21 = 7). So, Ann has the first 7 days of her fertility cycle to have intercourse.

The fertile phase begins the day after this infertile phase ends. In Ann's case, since the infertile phase ended on day 7, her fertile phase began on day 8. Her fertile phase will continue until she can successfully apply the rules used to determine when ovulation has passed and her infertile phase has begun.

Remember: The number 21 is used to determine the length of the infertile phase before ovulation because the greatest number of days that usually occur from ovulation to the end of the cycle is 16. The longest time that sperm may survive in fertile mucus is 5 days. Of course, 16 +

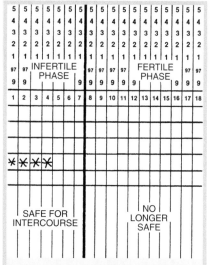

Fig. 24: Infertile phase before ovulation

Margo's previous six fertility cycles were 28 days in length. By subtracting 21 from 28, we see she has an infertile phase of 7 days. She can have intercourse from the first day of the fertility cycle up to and including cycle day 7 with a minimal chance of pregnancy. Since her infertile phase ends on cycle day 7, her fertile phase begins on cycle day 8. She would then abstain until ovulation has passed and her infertile phase has started.

5 = 21. Subtracting 21 from the shortest fertility cycle gives the number of days that are very safe for intercourse during the early part of the fertility cycle. In other words, by applying this rule you are counting back from the end of your cycle 16 days, then 5 more days. The number you get represents your infertile days early in the cycle, beginning with menstruation.

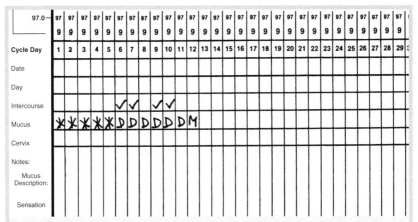

Fig. 25: Following the most conservative course: Putting the Menstrual Abstinence, Dry Day, and Early Mucus Rules together

Ellen experienced menstrual bleeding on cycle days 1–5. Abstinence was followed during these days. She then experienced dry days on cycle days 6–11. Ellen had intercourse the night of cycle day 6. This is recorded with a check mark (✔). Ellen used Kegels and bathed after intercourse that night. Because she experienced a dry day again on cycle day 7, she had intercourse again on that night. Cycle day 8 was dry again so Ellen could have had intercourse but chose not to. On cycle day 9 she had intercourse at night because it was a dry day. Ellen had intercourse again on the night of cycle day 10 because it was a dry day. She chose not to have intercourse on the night of cycle day 11. The fertile phase began on cycle day 12 because she observed non-wet mucus on this day. Ellen began to abstain and continued to do so until the infertile phase after ovulation began.

Don't forget, you can use this rule only if:

1. You can recall accurately when your last six cycles began

   or

2. You have kept a record of the beginning of your last six cycles

   or

3. You have been charting your fertility signs for six cycles.

To apply the 21 Day Rule, follow these requirements carefully:

1. Only use the shortest of the six most recent, consecutive cycles.

2. These must be normal ovulation cycles within the usual length for most women, which is 25–37 days long. If a woman recently stopped using any hormonal method of contraception, she must wait until she has experienced six normal fertility cycles after discontinuing the contraception to use the 21 Day Rule.

In practice, this rule is about 95–99 percent effective in avoiding pregnancy. The small 1–5 percent pregnancy rate is due to the fact that the rule does not take into account an unexpected early ovulation. *The warning sign of an early ovulation is cervical mucus.* If the woman is having intercourse whenever she wants during her infertile phase before ovulation, semen is present in the vagina. Therefore, she may not be able to see or feel the early ovulation signal of mucus and/or wet vaginal sensations. If she continues to have intercourse and ovulates earlier than usual, pregnancy can occur.

EXAMPLE: Joan's fertility cycles for the past two years have been 30–32 days long. Therefore, her infertile phase before ovulation is 9 days long (30 − 21 = 9). For the first 9 days of her cycle, Joan has had intercourse whenever she desired and has not become pregnant. In one fertility cycle Joan ovulated early. She was not aware of it because she was not watching her mucus sign, which would have been the signal for the early ovulation. She continued to have intercourse, and because fertile mucus was present, she became pregnant.

Short Cycle Calculations

If a woman's fertility cycles are usually less than 25 days long, she can use the 21 Day Rule to determine the length of her infertile phase before ovulation. For example, a woman's usual cycle lengths are 23 to 24 days. Her infertile phase before ovulation is therefore two days long (23 − 21 = 2). This is a very effective choice for women who would like to have at least a couple of days available for intercourse early in the menstrual cycle. There is probably about 1 to 5 percent chance of pregnancy using the 21 Day Rule with short cycles. A woman could also choose to be

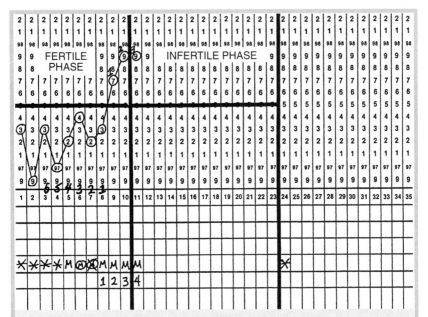

Fig. 26: The short cycle

Jade's previous 6 fertility cycles were 23–26 days in length. Since she normally experiences short fertility cycles, and is being most conservative, she does not give herself an infertile phase before ovulation by using the 21 Day Rule. Therefore, her fertile phase begins on the first day of her fertility cycle and ends when she can successfully apply the Last Wet Day and Thermal Shift Rules (see pages 104–109). In this example she had to abstain from cycle day 1 through cycle day 11. She could resume intercourse the night of cycle day 11 up to and including the end of her fertility cycle, day 23.

most conservative and begin her fertile phase on the first day of her cycle. In this case, abstinence would begin on the first day of menstruation.

Remember: Short cycles mean that ovulation takes place early in the cycle, a few days after the menstrual flow ends. Because of this, cervical mucus can be present during the menstrual flow. The bleeding makes observation of the mucus difficult if not impossible. If intercourse occurs and mucus is present, the sperm may be able to survive long enough to fertilize the egg at ovulation. The result is that for a woman with short cycles, pregnancy may occur from intercourse taking place during the first few days of her fertility cycle.

When a woman whose fertility cycle is short follows the most conservative approach, she has two instead of three phases to her fertility cycle—a fertile phase and an infertile phase after ovulation. *The first day of menstrual bleeding is the first day of the fertile phase.* The fertile phase ends and the infertile phase after ovulation begins when the Thermal Shift Rule and Last Wet Day Rule have been applied. (See pages 100–109.)

Decreasing the Possibility of Pregnancy Even Further

Is there a way of decreasing the chance of pregnancy during the infertile phase when using the 21 Day Rule? There is if the Dry Day Rule is followed. When a woman can calculate the length of her infertile phase before ovulation by using the 21 Day Rule, she also has the choice of using the Dry Day Rule. This way she will know if ovulation is going to occur early, because she will be able to recognize the early ovulation signals her body sends her: the earlier-than-usual appearance of cervical mucus and/or wet vaginal sensations. A woman can also choose to use either the Menstrual Abstinence Rule or the Menses Rule in combination with the 21 Day Rule. It is obvious that if a woman chooses to combine the 21 Day, Menstrual Abstinence, and Dry Day Rules together, she is deciding to be as conservative as possible.

One More Situation to Think About

What should a woman do if she does not have an accurate history of her most recent six fertility cycles or has just stopped using a hormonal method of birth control? In either of these situations, she does not have the proper information to use the 21 Day Rule. To be most conservative and safe, the woman should consider herself fertile from the first day of menstrual bleeding until her infertile phase after ovulation begins. Once she has six cycles recorded, the 21 Day rule can be used to determine the safe days early in the fertility cycle.

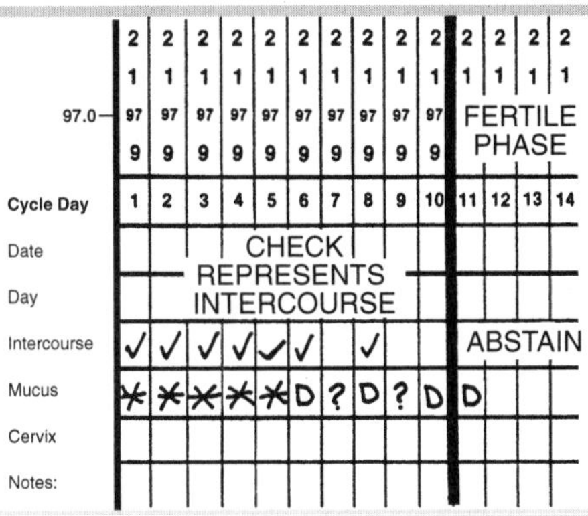

	2	2	2	2	2	2	2	2	2	2	2	2	2	2
	1	1	1	1	1	1	1	1	1	1	1	1	1	1
97.0 —	97	97	97	97	97	97	97	97	97	97	FERTILE			
	9	9	9	9	9	9	9	9	9	9	PHASE			
Cycle Day	1	2	3	4	5	6	7	8	9	10	11	12	13	14
Date			CHECK											
Day			REPRESENTS INTERCOURSE											
Intercourse	✓	✓	✓	✓	✓	✓		✓			ABSTAIN			
Mucus	✻	✻	✻	✻	✻	✻	D	?	D	?	D	D		
Cervix														
Notes:														

Fig. 27: The 21 Day Rule, Menses Rule, and Dry Day Rule

Naomi's last six cycles were 31 days long. Therefore, her infertile phase before ovulation is 10 days long (31 – 21 = 10). Because Naomi would like to minimize the chance of pregnancy while having intercourse before ovulation, she combined the use of the 21 Day, Menses, and Dry Day Rules. By following the Menses Rule, she could have intercourse anytime during the first 5 days of her cycle.

On cycle day 6 she experienced a dry day. By using the Dry Day Rule, she had intercourse on the evening of that day. She felt a wet vaginal sensation and saw some discharge in the morning so she abstained throughout cycle day 7 to allow time for semen to leave the vaginal area. On cycle day 8 she continued to abstain until she was sure the entire day was dry again. Because it was, she had intercourse on that evening.

She abstained on cycle day 9 again and because cycle day 10 was dry the entire day, it was still safe for intercourse. She didn't have intercourse on that day and found that on cycle day 11, she had another dry day. However, remember that she wants to follow the 21 Day Rule. According to the 21 day rule, her fertile phase had already begun on cycle day 11. This meant that even though she had a dry day on cycle day 11, she chose to follow the 21 Day Rule which was more conservative. Since her infertile phase ended on cycle day 10 according to the 21 Day Rule, her fertile phase began on cycle day 11 and so she began to abstain on that day.

However, some women find that waiting for six cycles to pass is unsatisfactory. They would like to have intercourse safely before ovulation even though they are not able to use the 21 Day Rule. These women choose to use the Dry Day and Menses Rules. In other words, they can have intercourse during the first five days of the cycle. Once the bleeding ends, they begin observing their cervical mucus. If mucus is not present throughout the entire day, and dry vaginal feelings are experienced, they can have intercourse on the night of each dry day. They then continue to use the Dry Day Rule until mucus production begins. Once mucus is observed and/or the vaginal feelings are no longer dry, the fertile phase has begun. Abstinence should be followed until the start of the infertile phase after ovulation.

NFP Rules Used to Determine the Infertile Phase after Ovulation

There are two rules that can be used to determine when the fertile phase ends and the infertile phase begins. One rule is used with mucus, the other with basal body temperature.

Last Wet Day Rule (Used with Mucus)

THE INFERTILE PHASE AFTER OVULATION BEGINS ON THE EVENING OF THE FOURTH DAY AFTER THE LAST DAY WET, SLIPPERY, AND STRETCHY MUCUS AND SLIPPERY, LUBRICATED VAGINAL SENSATIONS HAVE BEEN EXPERIENCED—WHICHEVER COMES LAST. (THIS IS ALSO KNOWN AS THE PEAK DAY RULE.)

As you know, at some point after ovulation, cervical mucus loses its slippery, stretchy, and wet quality, and the slippery, lubricated-feeling vaginal sensations go away. This is the way in which mucus sends a signal that ovulation has taken place. Slippery, stretchy mucus can no longer be observed, but sometimes the vaginal area still feels slippery and has a lubricated feeling to it for another day or two. The last day of slippery, lubricating vaginal sensations and/or wet, slippery, stretchy mucus (whichever is experienced last) has traditionally been called the "**peak day**" by many who work in the field of NFP. However, some argue that this name is confusing because the word "peak" typically means "the highest" or "the greatest" and the peak day is NOT the day of the most slippery, stretchy mucus or the greatest amount of mucus. It is not the day of the most slippery vaginal sensation either. It may not even be the day of greatest fertility. It can be, but that may not be true for every woman. So, instead of "peak day" we will use the term "**last wet day**" to mean simply the *last* day that a woman observes signs of fertility in her mucus and vaginal sensations.

Can the last day be identified in advance? No, unfortunately it can't be predicted in advance. The last wet day can only be identified after it has passed. For example, a woman can experience slippery, stretchy, and wet mucus and slippery, lubricating vaginal sensations from Monday through Friday; then on Saturday her mucus is no longer wet and stretchy and her vaginal sensations are not longer wet and slippery as well. This means that Friday was her last wet day.

One more word about vaginal sensations: As you have probably noticed, we continuously reinforce paying attention to vaginal sensations. Remember that these sensations reflect the quality of the mucus present. Wet mucus

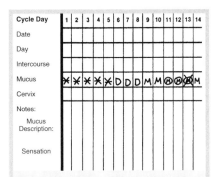

Fig. 28: Identifying the last wet day

Joanne has recorded 5 days of menstrual bleeding. Once the bleeding ended, she began observing for mucus. On cycle days 6, 7, and 8, because no mucus was observed and a dry vaginal feeling was experienced, these days were recorded as dry days. On cycle days 9 and 10 she experienced a pasty, sticky mucus with a dry vaginal feeling.

Joanne began producing wet, slippery, and stretchy mucus on cycle day 11. This type of mucus continued until cycle day 13. On cycle day 14 she noticed that her wet, slippery vaginal feelings and slippery mucus were no longer present. Joanne's vaginal area felt dry and she observed sticky, pasty mucus. At this point she was able to go back to cycle day 13, her last day of slippery, stretchy mucus and slippery vaginal feelings, and mark it as her last wet day. Placing an **X** through the circled **M** represents the last wet day for that cycle.

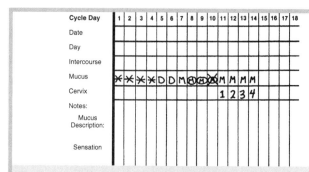

Fig. 29: The Last Wet Day Rule

Marlene no longer experienced slippery vaginal sensations on cycle day 11, and her mucus felt less wet and slippery than it had on cycle days 8, 9, and 10. Because of this she could mark cycle day 10, the last wet and slippery mucus day, as her last wet day. Marlene could then apply the Last Wet Day Rule because she experienced 4 days of sticky, pasty mucus and sticky vaginal feelings in a row after her last wet day. Her infertile phase after ovulation began on the evening of cycle day 14.

causes a wet vaginal feeling; slippery mucus causes a slippery feeling; and a total absence of mucus or sticky, pasty, and crumbly mucus causes a dry or sticky vaginal feeling.

If you feel a wet, slippery feeling but don't see any more slippery mucus, your last wet day has not yet occurred. You have experienced *the last wet day* only when both the mucus and vaginal feelings are no longer wet, slippery, and lubricating.

Once the last wet day is determined, the rule can be applied.

Remember, ovulation can occur any time from up to three days before the last wet day to one day after the last wet day. Waiting until the evening of the fourth day to resume intercourse provides sufficient time for the release and life span of the egg. When the infertile phase begins, you no longer need to observe your mucus.

It's not the last wet day! Occasionally a woman experiences the reappearance of slippery, stretchy, and wet mucus after she has identified what she believed to be her last wet day. She will know it was not her real last wet day because instead of having four sticky, pasty, and crumbly mucus and/or

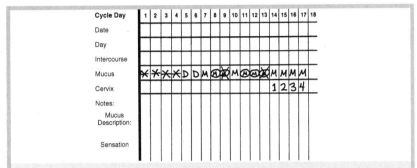

Fig. 30: Identifying the true last wet day

Ruth thought her last wet day occurred on cycle day 9, since on cycle day 10 she experienced a sticky, pasty mucus with dry vaginal sensations. However, while waiting for the four days to pass, she noticed a reappearance of wet, slippery mucus on cycle day 11 and her vaginal sensations felt slippery. She realized that either she had made an error in identifying her last wet day or perhaps she was ovulating later than usual.

Ruth continued to abstain and waited until her wet, slippery mucus production stopped and her vaginal sensations were no longer slippery and wet. She then identified a last wet day on cycle day 13. This time she was correct, because she then experienced sticky, pasty mucus days with dry vaginal sensations for four days in a row. Therefore, according to the Last Wet Day Rule, her infertile phase began the evening of cycle day 17.

dry days in a row, wet and/or stretchy, slippery mucus reappears. If this happens, abstinence should be continued until the real last wet day is identified and the vaginal sensations and mucus no longer feel slippery and wet and the mucus is no longer stretchy for four days in a row.

There are two common reasons for this happening. First, and most commonly, a woman makes a mistake in identifying her last wet day. This more commonly occurs when someone is just learning about her mucus changes.

The greater a woman's experience with mucus observations, the less likely the possibility that she will incorrectly identify her last wet day. There is another reason, however, why a woman might think she has experienced her last wet day when this isn't the case. Ovulation can be delayed. A delay in ovulation can cause wet, slippery mucus and wet, slippery vaginal sensations to come and go until the egg is finally released. These situations need not be a problem if two key points are remembered:

1. Always wait until the evening of the fourth sticky, pasty, and crumbly mucus and/or dry day after the last wet day to resume intercourse. Vaginal feelings must be dry or sticky during these four days.

2. Always wait to resume intercourse until the Thermal Shift Rule is applied. (See below.)

The temperature pattern can help you greatly if these situations occur, since the last wet day usually occurs around the same time as the thermal shift, often within one to two days before the shift happens. This means that the beginning of the infertile phase is often the same when the Thermal Shift and Last Wet Day Rules are applied. *When this is not the case, the more conservative rule must be followed before resuming intercourse.*

For example, if you have applied the Thermal Shift Rule and it gives you an infertile phase beginning Wednesday evening, and the Last Wet Day Rule gives you an infertile phase beginning on Tuesday evening, intercourse should not begin until Wednesday evening.

Thermal Shift Rule (Used with Basal Body Temperature)

THE INFERTILE PHASE AFTER OVULATION BEGINS ON THE NIGHT OF THE THIRD CONSECUTIVE TEMPERATURE RECORDED ABOVE THE COVERLINE.

The Thermal Shift Rule is the rule that is applied to the basal body temperature. It is called the "Thermal Shift Rule" because to use it you must measure a shift or rise in basal body temperature, from the low temperatures experienced before ovulation to the higher temperatures experienced around the time of ovulation. The basal body temperatures will rise usually 0.3°–1.0°F or 0.15°–0.6°C higher than the low tempera-

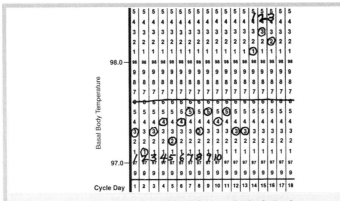

Fig. 31: The Thermal Shift Rule

Ann's temperature shifted to 98.1°F on cycle day 14. To draw the coverline, we look at the first ten temperatures. Next, we find the highest of the ten temperatures. In this case it is 97.5°F. Finally, by adding $1/10$ of a degree to 97.5°F, we can draw the coverline at 97.6°F. Waiting for three temperatures in a row to be recorded above the coverline gives us an infertile phase beginning on the evening of cycle day 16.

tures recorded up to that point. This usually happens the same day or one to two days after the egg is released.

To apply the Thermal Shift Rule, follow these steps:

1. Each morning, take your BBT as described in Chapter 5. After you have recorded temperatures from cycle days 1–10, look at these temperatures and locate the highest one you have recorded.

2. Draw a line across your chart that is just 0.1°F or 0.05°C above the highest temperature you recorded during the first ten days of the fertility cycle. This line is called the **coverline**.

3. Continue to take your basal body temperature. At some point, the temperatures will rise above the coverline.

4. Once this happens, your infertile phase after ovulation will begin on the night of the third consecutive temperature recorded above the coverline.

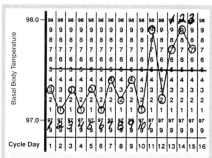

Fig. 32: Identifying the true thermal shift

Maria's temperature shifted to 97.9°F on cycle day 11. The coverline was drawn at 97.5°F, which is $1/10$ of a degree above the highest of the first ten low temperatures. As you can see, the temperature dropped back down below the coverline on cycle day 12. Therefore, we have to wait until the true shift in temperature takes place to determine the beginning of the infertile phase.

Maria's temperature rises again on cycle day 13. We know this is the true thermal shift because the temperature stays above the line for three days in a row. Therefore, in this example the infertile phase begins on the evening of cycle day 15.

It is important to wait for three days of high temperatures to resume intercourse because ovulation may not occur until the day after the rise in temperature. To be most conservative, let's say this is when ovulation happens in a particular cycle. The egg will only live up to 24 hours unless it is fertilized. Waiting to resume intercourse until the evening of the third day allows sufficient time for the release and life span of one, and perhaps two, eggs. If an egg is no longer present, there can be no pregnancy!

Caution: If any one of the three temperatures falls on or below the coverline, it can be a sign that ovulation has not yet taken place. Therefore, wait until the temperatures rise back above the coverline and then apply the three-day count again.

Occasionally, around the time of ovulation, you may observe a rise in temperature and assume it is your thermal shift. However, instead of remaining above the coverline for three consecutive days, the temperature may fall back on or below it. Therefore, the temperature rise was for a reason other than ovulation. This is called a **false high rise** (Figure 33). A false high rise can be caused by oversleeping one day or by experiencing one of the situations discussed in Chapter 7 that can cause an unusual temperature rise. False high rises, as we have stated, cannot be used when applying the Thermal Shift Rule. Always use only those high temperatures that reflect accurate normal basal body temperatures.

A false high temperature can also occur early in the fertility cycle. For example, let's say a woman's temperature rises abnormally high on cycle day 7 because she had a restless night's sleep. The temperature goes back to its normal low level on cycle day 8. If this happens, the high temperature on cycle day 7 would not be used to determine the coverline. Instead, it would be thrown out (or ignored). The remaining nine low temperatures would be used to draw the coverline.

Some women experience high temperatures during menstruation because

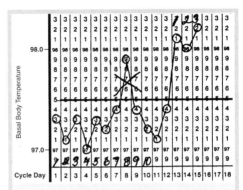

Fig. 33: False high rise

Jane's temperature rises on cycle day 8. Because the rise had taken place in the early part of Jane's fertility cycle, before she usually experiences her thermal shift, she knew this rise was probably not her real thermal shift. She also overslept that morning and took her temperature a couple of hours later than usual.

On cycle day 9, the temperature dropped again, proving that the BBT on day 8 represented a false high rise. Jane continued to take her temperature and found that it shifted on cycle day 13. She drew her coverline $1/10$ of a degree above the highest of the first ten temperatures of her cycle before the thermal shift. Since the temperature on cycle day 8 was unusually high, it would not be used to draw the coverline, even though it was counted as one of the ten temperatures recorded.

progesterone, a hormone that produces heat, is probably still affecting the temperatures. This does not happen often, but it is possible. By the time bleeding ends, the temperatures have returned to low levels again. However, this doe not affect a woman's ability to apply the Thermal Shift Rule correctly. For example, if the first three temperatures of a

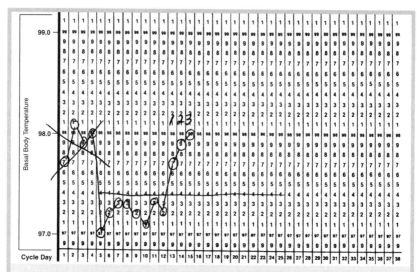

Fig. 34: High temperatures during bleeding

Angela experienced temperatures ranging from 97.7–98.1°F during the first four days of her menstrual period. Her temperature went down to 97.0°F on cycle day 5 and continued in the low range through cycle day 10. The highest temperature recorded during cycle days 5 through 10 was 97.3°F. Angela drew her coverline at 97.4°F and waited until she experienced three consecutive temperatures recorded above the coverline. This happened on cycle days 13, 14, and 15. Her infertile phase after ovulation began on the evening of cycle day 15.

woman's cycle are high, she would "throw them out" and not use them to determine the coverline. Her temperature returns to a low level on cycle day 4 and continues low through cycle day 10. She would use the temperatures from days 4–10 to draw her coverline.

Earlier-Than-Usual Ovulation

When using the Thermal Shift Rule, always be aware of the possibility of early ovulation. A woman who ovulates early in her cycle will experience a thermal shift before ten temperatures have been recorded. If she is checking her mucus and vaginal sensations, she will notice that both become wet and slippery. When the temperature goes up, the woman

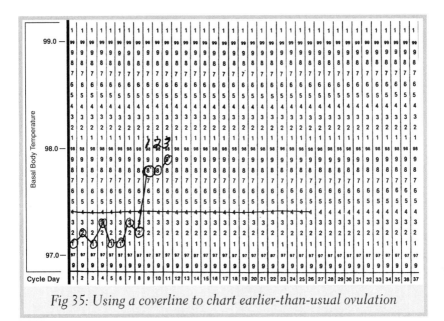

Fig 35: Using a coverline to chart earlier-than-usual ovulation

should draw a coverline 0.1°F above the highest temperatures recorded up to that point. Once this is done, the Thermal Shift Rule can be applied.

For example, if you experience a thermal shift on cycle day 9, draw a coverline 0.1°F or 0.05°C above the highest normal low temperature recorded from cycle day 1–8. Once the coverline is drawn, continue to take your temperature. Once three consecutive temperatures have been recorded above the coverline, the infertile phase after ovulation has begun.

TO REVIEW

✤ Find the highest normal low temperature recorded during the first ten days of the fertility cycle.

✤ Draw the coverline 0.1° F or 0.05° C above the highest of the ten temperatures.

✤ Wait for three days in a row of high temperatures above the coverline.

✦ The evening of the third day of high temperatures is the beginning of the infertile phase after ovulation, and intercourse can be resumed until the next menstrual flow begins.

✦ You can put your thermometer away after the beginning of the infertile phase.

Charting your basal body temperature is an accurate way of determining that you have ovulated and are no longer able to become pregnant. Remember that the temperature rises around the time of ovulation. Therefore, it makes sense to use the temperature shift in combination with the changes in cervical mucus in order to be as accurate as possible in determining the beginning of the infertile time after ovulation. Another advantage in using the basal body temperature is

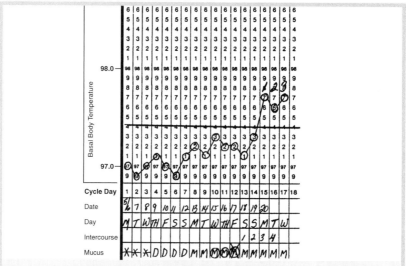

Fig. 36: Combining the Last Wet Day and Thermal Shift Rules
(Always use the more conservative rule)

Sheri applied both the Last Wet Day Rule and Thermal Shift Rule. The Last Wet Day Rule gave an infertile phase beginning on the evening of cycle day 16. However, the Thermal Shift Rule gave an infertile phase beginning on the evening of cycle day 17. To be safe, Sheri used the more conservative rule—in this case the Thermal Shift Rule—and her infertile phase began the evening of cycle day 17.

that it can help you make sure you have identified the last wet day properly. When you apply both the Thermal Shift Rule and the Last Wet Day Rule, remember to follow the more conservative rule.

Another example of applying the Thermal Shift and Last Wet Day Rules together can be found in Figure 36.

Summary of the Infertile and Fertile Times of the Fertility Cycle

The Infertile Phase Before Ovulation includes:

1. the menstrual flow

2. days that are dry (mucus is not present and there is a dry vaginal sensation)

3. days in which the cervix is low, firm, and closed

4. low basal body temperatures, with the possible exception of a few higher temperatures which may occur during the menstrual flow

The Fertile Phase includes:

1. all mucus days until the Last Wet Day Rule is applied

2. days in which the cervix is higher in the vaginal canal and is soft and open

3. the rising of the basal body temperature from low levels to high levels until the Thermal Shift Rule is applied

The Infertile Phase After Ovulation includes:

1. days when mucus is pasty, sticky, and crumbly and/or days that are completely dry (note that as previously discussed, some women experience a wet discharge shortly before menstrual bleeding begins. This isn't a fertile type mucus but a fluid that comes from the lining of the uterus as it begins to go through changes that will lead to menstrual bleeding).

2. days in which the cervix is low, firm, and closed

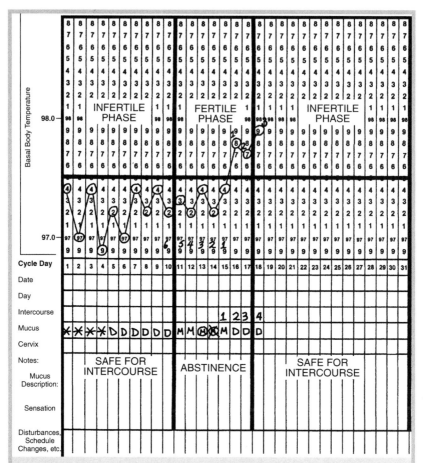

Fig. 37: The infertile and fertile times of the fertility cycle

Angela's last six fertility cycles were 31 days in length. Therefore, according to the 21 Day Rule, her infertile phase before ovulation is 10 days long. (31 – 21 = 10) Depending upon how conservative a method of NFP she wants to use, she can use the 21 Day Rule to guide her in having intercourse before her fertile phase begins and have intercourse whenever she desires during that phase. She could be more conservative and use the 21 Day Rule with the Menses Rule (first 5 days). Her fertile phase began on cycle day 11 as determined by the 21 Day Rule. She began to abstain on that day.

By application of the Thermal Shift Rule and Last Wet Day Rule, she could resume intercourse on the night of cycle day 18. She could then have intercourse whenever she wanted up to and including cycle day 31.

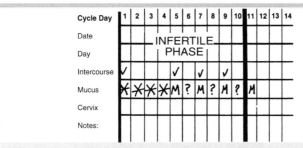

Fig. 38: The basic infertile mucus pattern

Cheryl had observed the same type of mucus every day for 6 days after her menstrual period ended. Because she felt she had gained the experience needed to be confident with her mucus observations, she used the days of non-changing mucus (or her basic infertile pattern) as though they were dry days. Her fertile phase began on cycle day 11 because her mucus changed. It became slightly wet, indicating the approach of ovulation.

Note that there are several "?"s in the mucus boxes on the days after Cheryl had intercourse. This is because she had wet discharge that could have been mucus or semen. She thus had to abstain for 24 hours to see if her basic infertile pattern returned before having intercourse again.

The Basic Infertile Mucus Pattern

We discussed the concept of the basic infertile pattern (BIP) when we first described normal mucus patterns in Chapter 5. This is the pattern by which a woman's body reveals to her that she is probably experiencing an infertile time before ovulation. For many women, the BIP is one of dry days. However, there are some women who always see mucus as soon as the menstrual flow ends, instead of experiencing dry days. These women experience the same type of mucus every day during the infertile phase before ovulation. The mucus doesn't feel wet or slippery and the vaginal sensations are either dry or sticky. This situation of daily non-changing mucus and vaginal sensations that do not have any classic fertile characteristics is the basic infertile pattern for these women. Since there are no dry days during the infertile phase before ovulation, the Dry Day Rule is applied to the BIP of non-changing mucus and vaginal sensations. In other words, because the woman doesn't have dry days but instead has non-changing mucus, the non-changing mucus days are used as though they were dry, no-mucus days.

Therefore, for women who never experience dry days, intercourse may occur on the night of any day with non-changing mucus and non-changing vaginal sensations.

These women must be careful to be on the lookout for any change from their basic infertile pattern. *If the mucus or vaginal feelings change in any way, it may mean that ovulation is approaching.* If the mucus does change, and/or the vaginal sensations change, the fertile phase has started and abstinence must begin.

Caution: A woman may need to observe her mucus for two or more fertility cycles to develop the experience necessary to use this rule.

If you wish to use the natural family planning rules well, it is important to do the following:

* ❖ observe your fertility signs accurately

* ❖ chart your fertility signs and changes accurately

* ❖ follow the rules as they have been explained

Sympto-Thermal Method Choices

As we explained in Chapter 2, the sympto-thermal method of natural family planning combines observation of mucus, basal body temperature, and other fertility signs. The basic choices for couples using this method are:

BEFORE OVULATION

1. A couple can abstain during menstrual bleeding (Menstrual Abstinence Rule)

   or

   have intercourse during the first five days of the fertility cycle if ovulation occurred the previous cycle (Menses Rule, page 91). A couple can also have intercourse on the night of a dry day (Dry Day Rule, page 87) or a non-changing mucus day (for women who have a basic infertile pattern of non-changing mucus). These rules can be used with or without the 21 Day Rule (page 93).

2. The fertile phase begins when:

   – any type of mucus and/or wet, slippery vaginal sensations are experienced (Early Mucus Rule, page 90); or

   – the 21 Day Rule is applied (page 93)

   If a woman is using both the Early Mucus and 21 Day Rules together, the more conservative rule should be followed.

   If a woman usually has a basic infertile pattern of non-changing mucus, her fertile phase would begin whenever she experiences any kind of change in her mucus and/or vaginal sensations.

AFTER OVULATION

3. The Last Wet Day (page 100) and Thermal Shift (page 104) Rules should be applied and the more conservative rule followed.

For an example of a fertility chart in which all of these rules have been followed see Figure 39 on the next page.

Using the Cervical Mucus Method to Prevent Pregnancy

Some women cannot or do not want to observe their basal body temperature and instead choose to follow cervical mucus changes to prevent pregnancy. Though this book is primarily devoted to discussing the sympto-thermal method, we'd like to introduce this family planning option because use of cervical mucus to prevent pregnancy is an effective method of NFP. If you would like to use the cervical mucus method, we advise reading *The Ovulation Method* by Dr. John J. Billings, and attending a cervical mucus method program in your area. There is also a Billings Method website you can access at www.billingsmethod.com.

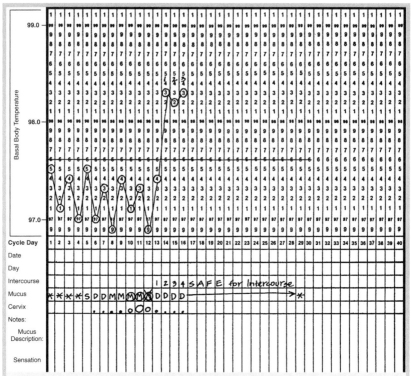

Fig. 39: All the infertile phase after ovulation rules

Kim observed her mucus, cervix, and basal body temperature, and by apply-ing all the rules saw that her infertile phase began on the evening of cycle day 16. Since her menstrual cycle was 30 days long, she could safely have inter-course from the evening of the 16th day up to and including cycle day 30. Dur-ing these days she no longer needed to observe her fertility signs.

Cervical Mucus Method Rules

The most conservative rules to use with mucus observations are:

Rule Number 1—The Menstrual Abstinence Rule

INTERCOURSE SHOULD BE AVOIDED DURING MENSTRUAL BLEEDING.

This rule exists primarily because of the possibility that ovulation could occur close to the time menstruation ends, and during menstruation a woman can find it difficult to accurately assess cervical mucus and vaginal sensations.

It is also important to note that a woman may assume she is menstruating but instead be experiencing bleeding for various other reasons, such as ovulation, a hormone imbalance, or a problem in the reproductive organs. If ovulation is occurring or is about to occur and a couple has intercourse, pregnancy can result. (If a woman experiences bleeding that she feels may not be menstrual bleeding, it is important to discuss this with her health-care provider.)

OPTION TO RULE NUMBER 1—THE MENSES RULE: Intercourse can take place during the first five days of the fertility cycle if a woman has successfully applied the Last Wet Day Rule the previous cycle and the cycle appeared normal for her.

Rule Number 2—The Dry Day Rule

INTERCOURSE CAN OCCUR THE NIGHT OF ANY DRY DAY
DURING THE INFERTILE PHASE BEFORE OVULATION.

This is the same Dry Day Rule explained in our discussion of the sympto-thermal method rules.

OPTION TO RULE NUMBER 2: If the day after intercourse is dry the entire day, abstinence does not need to be followed and intercourse can once again occur on that evening.

Rule Number 3—The Early Mucus Rule

THE FERTILE PHASE ALWAYS BEGINS ON THE FIRST DAY ANY
TYPE OF MUCUS IS OBSERVED AND/OR WET, SLIPPERY VAGINAL
SENSATIONS ARE EXPERIENCED...

...unless a woman's basic infertile pattern is non-changing, non-wet mucus with dry or sticky vaginal sensations. In this case, the fertile phase begins on the first day on which any change from the basic infertile mucus pattern is observed and felt. For the woman who has dry days after her period ends, her fertile phase begins even if the sticky, pasty, and crumbly mucus is present. This is still an indication that a woman has probably entered her fertile time. Remember that although this mucus is typically the infertile type, when it is seen before ovulation after dry days have been experienced, it could be a signal that wet, slippery, and stretchy, fertile mucus is starting to be produced in the cervix but hasn't yet traveled down to the vaginal opening where it can be seen. Consequently, intercourse at this time could result in pregnancy.

What is the possibility of pregnancy when intercourse takes place on the days on which sticky, pasty, and crumbly mucus is observed? The answer to this question is not known at the present time. Some sources state that the chances are very small. However, an actual pregnancy rate based on couples having intercourse when this kind of mucus is present before ovulation has not been determined. Therefore, if you want the most conservative approach, abstinence should be followed every day beginning with the first day that any type of mucus appears, and continuing until the fertile phase has ended.

Rule Number 4—The Last Wet Day Rule

THE INFERTILE PHASE AFTER OVULATION BEGINS ON THE EVENING OF THE FOURTH DAY AFTER THE LAST DAY WET, SLIPPERY, AND STRETCHY MUCUS AND SLIPPERY, LUBRICATED VAGINAL SENSATIONS HAVE BEEN EXPERIENCED—WHICHEVER COMES LAST. (THIS IS ALSO KNOWN AS THE PEAK DAY RULE.)

This rule is used to determine the beginning of the infertile phase after ovulation.

Applying the Sympto-Thermal NFP Rules

Before you begin charting your own cycles, you might want to carefully review Alicia's chart on the next page. Also, a full explanation of the NFP rules she followed during her cycle and why can be found on pages 119–121.

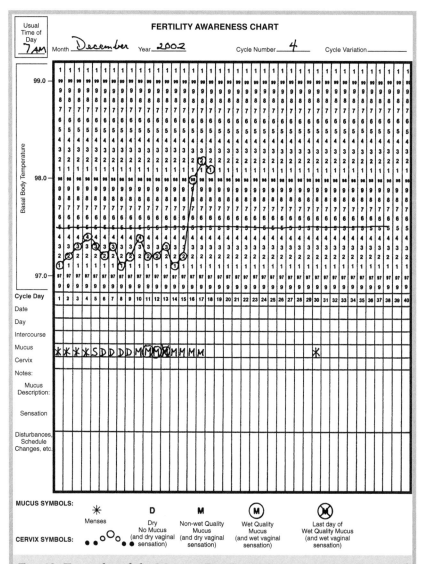

Fig. 40: Examples of the Menses, Dry Day, Mucus, Last Wet Day, and Thermal Shift Rules

Alicia has been recording her mucus and temperature for three cycles. Before these three cycles, she had never kept a record of her cycle lengths, but guesses they were about 28 days in length. Her last three cycles have ranged from 28–32 days in length. She usually takes her temperature at *(cont'd...)*

7:00 A.M. Last cycle, Alicia knew she ovulated because she had a rise in her temperature and could apply the Thermal Shift Rule. She also experienced a last wet day and applied the Last Wet Day Rule.

1.   Could Alicia have intercourse during menstrual bleeding? Yes. Since Alicia applied the Last Wet Day and Thermal Shift Rules the previous fertility cycle, she knows the bleeding she experienced this cycle is a true menstrual period. Therefore, she could have intercourse during cycle days 1–5 (Menses Rule).

2.   Could Alicia apply the 21 Day Rule to determine the length of her infertile time before ovulation? No, because she does not have accurate knowledge of her cycle lengths for the last six cycles.

3.   If Alicia had intercourse on cycle day 5 (which is also a dry day) could she have intercourse on cycle day 6? Yes, if she did not observe any cervical mucus and then had dry vaginal sensations throughout cycle day 6, then intercourse could take place on the night of cycle day 6. If Alicia experienced a dry day again on cycle day 7, she could have intercourse that night. If she had intercourse and cycle day 8 was dry, she could have intercourse again on the night of cycle day 8. Remember, if Alicia had experienced a vaginal discharge on a day after intercourse, she would have to abstain for 24 hours to know whether the discharge was semen, mucus, or both. If, after the 24 hours of abstinence, she experienced a dry day again, she could have intercourse that night.

4.   When does the fertile phase begin? It begins on cycle day 10, since this is when Alicia experienced mucus. Though it wasn't wet mucus and she did not have a wet and/or slippery vaginal sensation, she knows that wet mucus could be up in the cervix. She also knows wet mucus could take a day to travel down to the vaginal opening, where she could see it.

5.   When does the fertile phase end? To determine this, the last wet day needs to be identified. This was on cycle day 13. Remember, the last wet day is the last day of wet, stretchy mucus and wet, slippery vaginal sensations. To apply the Last Wet Day Rule, Alicia must continue to abstain until four days of non-wet mucus and/or dry days with sticky and/or dry vaginal sensations after the last wet day. The fertile phase ends on the night of the fourth day after the last wet day, which in this case is cycle day 17. Intercourse can be resumed on the night of the fourth day and continue until the end of the cycle.

Alicia should also apply the Thermal Shift Rule to know when the fertile phase has ended. To do this, she first needs to draw the coverline 0.1°F or 0.05°C above the highest temperature recorded during the first ten days of her cycle. Once this is done, she must be sure she has recorded *(cont'd...)*

three consecutive temperatures that are above the coverline. The infertile phase begins on the night of the third high temperature recorded above the coverline. In this case, the night of the third high temperature was recorded on cycle day 18.

The Last Wet Day Rule shows that the infertile phase begins on the night of cycle day 17, but the Thermal Shift Rule shows that the infertile phase begins on the night of cycle day 18. Therefore, to be most conservative, the infertile phase begins on the night of cycle day 18. Intercourse can be resumed on this night and can continue any day, any time, until the menses begins again. Alicia can stop observing her fertility signs on cycle day 19 until the next cycle begins. When Alicia has recorded six cycles, she can choose to use the 21 Day Rule with or without checking her mucus.

When Can You Begin Using These Rules to Prevent Pregnancy?

During the first cycle of observing and charting, you may be able to use these rules to determine the infertile phase after ovulation. However, this can be done *only* if you feel you have observed and recorded your fertility signs carefully and applied the Last Wet Day Rule, Thermal Shift Rule, or both rules correctly. If you are not confident with using the method, wait at least another fertility cycle, until you are more comfortable with your own fertility pattern, before you apply these rules. You must be confident that you are following the instructions for checking and charting properly, and applying the rules correctly, before assuming you are no longer fertile and resuming intercourse.

YOUR NOTES

10

Special Circumstances: The Later Years, Breastfeeding, Illnesses, Etc.

It is not uncommon for us to make plans that have to be changed at the last minute. Yet the change need not ruin our day if we make room for it to happen.

This is true of the fertility cycle. Natural family planning can be used successfully with the normal ovulatory cycle, and if something happens to cause a change in the cycle or the patterns of the fertility signs, the NFP rules can still be followed to prevent pregnancy.

Any situations that cause a change in your fertility cycle or patterns of fertility signs are called special circumstances.

If special circumstances occur, you can often continue to use fertility signs successfully to prevent pregnancy by knowing what to look for and by using the special circumstances rules explained in this chapter.

Special circumstances include

+ fever

+ breastfeeding

+ stress

+ ovarian cyst

+ previous birth control pill use

+ change in exercise regimen

+ change in diet

✤ travel

✤ illness

✤ perimenopause

We will save a detailed discussion of each of these different types of special circumstances until later in the chapter. First, we will outline some basic points about special circumstances and the use of NFP. Learning how to use NFP in special circumstances is, for many, the most difficult aspect of NFP. Therefore, we will help you understand how to deal with them by discussing only a few of the more common special circumstances. Later, we will explore some of the other special circumstances and fertility sign patterns.

Special circumstances can be separated into two categories:

1. Circumstances that change the normal pattern of your BBT and/or cervical mucus and vaginal sensations. These include circumstances that cause the BBT to be abnormally high, such as an illness causing a fever, or circumstances that cause the cervical mucus to have an abnormal appearance, such as a vaginal infection.

2. Circumstances that stop ovulation from happening for a while or cause an earlier- or later-than-usual ovulation. These can include just about anything and everything in life. In fact, all of the special circumstances we previously listed could affect the time of ovulation.

The most common circumstances that might affect your BBT pattern are typical life situations, such as an everyday cold, the flu, or any health problem that produces a fever. The BBT can rise due to other life situations as well, such as going through a stressful time in your life that disrupts your normal sleep pattern, or being in the perimenopausal time of your life and experiencing an increase in body temperature at different times of the day and/or night.

You need not stop charting your BBT to prevent pregnancy during a cycle in which you have a fever or experience high temperatures for any other reason. If you see your temperature rising higher than usual or rising earlier than expected (whether or not you are feeling ill), you need to watch this unexpected temperature change carefully. If the temperature rises above 99°F as measured with a BBT thermometer, it is important to continue taking your temperature with a fever thermometer once in the morning and once in the evening until the fever is no longer present. You should switch to using a fever thermometer, since it measures the body temperature up to 108°F. The markings on the basal body thermometer only go up to 100°F. You will not be able to know how high your fever actually is if you use your basal body thermometer. The basal body thermometer could even break if you attempt to use it to measure unusually high temperatures.

The unusually high temperature should be recorded on the fertility awareness chart in a special way each day it is present. If the temperature is higher than the temperatures printed on the chart (the chart goes up to 99°F), a line should be drawn from the last normal basal body temperature to the very top of the chart (Figure 41). Each day the temperature remains "off the chart," it should be recorded in the "Notes" column. If your BBT is high because of a fever, it will, of course, return to normal when the fever is gone. If your BBT is high for other life reasons, it is difficult to know when it will return to normal. If the temperature rise is due to stress, the determining factor is the way in which the stress is dealt with and how long it will take the body to recover from the effects of stress. If the temperature rise is due to perimenopause, there is no way of predicting when the BBT will return to normal. Regardless of the cause of a high BBT, use of the BBT thermometer should be resumed when the body temperature returns to normal.

When the body temperature rises due to a fever or other life situation, one of three situations may occur during the fertility cycle:

1. Ovulation will occur as usual and the fertility cycle will be its usual length.

2. Ovulation will occur later than usual and the fertility cycle will be longer than its usual length.

3. Ovulation will not occur at all for a while and bleeding may or may not be experienced. Even if bleeding takes place around the time you would expect to see menstrual bleeding, do not consider this a true menstrual period. Some women experience bleeding very much like a menstrual period when they do not ovulate. This is called anovulatory bleeding. The bleeding could also be occurring because ovulation is taking place at that time. In either case, it is not safe to have intercourse.

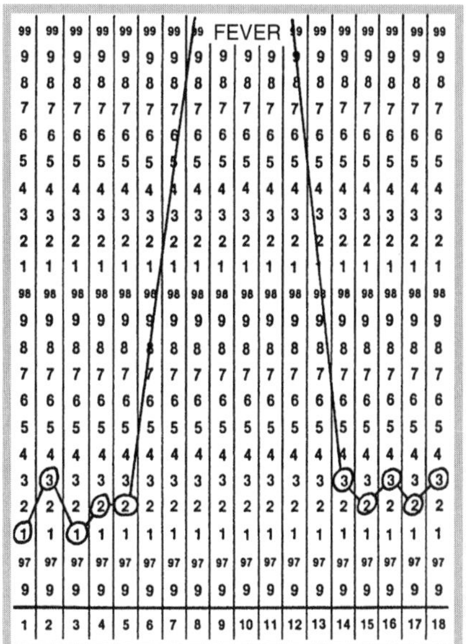

Ovulation on Time

When something causes an abnormally high BBT during the time of ovulation, a thermal shift cannot be seen. However, if you ovulated, you will know it because, once the fever is gone, the basal body temperature will drop back down to the high temperatures you normally experience after ovulation.

Fig. 41: Charting a fever

Sue began observing and recording her basal body temperature from the first day of her fertility cycle. From cycle day 6 through cycle day 13 she experienced a fever above 99.1°F. She noted the presence of a fever on her chart. When the fever went away, she continued to observe and record her basal body temperature.

Observe your mucus during the abnormally high temperatures. If the Last Wet Day Rule can be applied, you can follow this rule to determine when the infertile phase has begun. However, if you are not confident using this rule alone, you will have to continue to abstain until you can accurately apply the BBT rule as well.

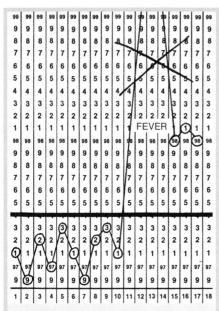

Fig. 42: Fever during the time of ovulation

Alice experienced a fever from cycle day 11 through cycle day 14. Once the fever subsided, her basal body temperature was at the normal (but elevated) level experienced after ovulation. This indicated that ovulation had taken place at some point during the fever. To determine the infertile phase, she applied the Thermal Shift Rule. She drew a coverline above the first ten normal low temperatures recorded before the fever. She skipped over the fever and then used the first three normal high temperatures she recorded after the fever to determine when her infertile phase after ovulation began. These were recorded on cycle days 15, 16, and 17. Therefore, her infertile phase began on the night of cycle day 17.

Late or Delayed Ovulation

Ovulation may be delayed during a life situation that elevates temperature, such as those previously described. A delayed ovulation is one that happens later than usual. With a delayed ovulation the thermal shift may not be seen until a few days or up to a few weeks later than expected. If ovulation did not occur during the time of abnormally high temperatures, once the fever subsides, the temperatures will return to the normal low level experienced before ovulation. In this situation, the woman should continue to take her BBT until the Thermal Shift Rule can be applied (Figure 43).

No Ovulation

No ovulation is called *anovulation*. You may not ovulate at all during the time of a life situation that causes abnormally high temperatures, such as those described above. When ovulation does not take place, it makes sense that the pat-

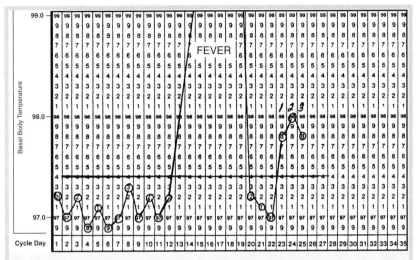

Fig. 43: Fever and delayed ovulation

Elisa usually has fertility cycles ranging from 28–32 days. During a cycle when she was ill, she experienced ovulation later than was usual for her. This was seen by the fact that when her fever subsided on cycle day 20, her basal body temperature was still in the low range that is experienced before ovulation. On cycle day 23 her temperature finally shifted and she was then able to apply the Thermal Shift Rule to determine her infertile phase. She drew a coverline over the highest of the first ten temperatures of her cycle and then skipped over the fever. Once the fever subsided, she continued to take her BBT. When three consecutive temperatures were recorded above the coverline, she could determine the beginning of her infertile phase, which was on the evening of cycle day 25.

terns of fertility signs will no longer be the ones normally seen with ovulation. Let's take a brief moment to review some facts about ovulation and hormones before looking at some examples of fertility sign changes during a time of anovulation.

If we divide the cycle into two parts for the purpose of this discussion, we have the part before ovulation and the part after ovulation. As you have learned, the part before ovulation is under the control of the hormone estrogen. Estrogen is produced in increasing amounts as a result of an egg maturing. This hormone reaches a very high level when the egg is just about ready to leave the ovary. After the egg leaves the ovary, the hormone progesterone is produced in increasingly high amounts and is in control after ovulation, even though a good amount of estrogen is still being made.

Without these hormones reaching the high levels that occur with ovulation, a woman cannot expect to see certain changes in her fertility signs. For example, without a high level of estrogen, cervical mucus never becomes the typical very stretchy, wet mucus you would experience when you ovulate and your vaginal sensations never reach a very wet, slippery state. Some estrogen is usually being produced by the ovary throughout a woman's reproductive lifetime and eggs can grow for a few days and then stop growing. When this happens, the mucus can change at different times and even feel somewhat wet, slippery and stretchy. However, it will never change to the very wet, stretchy, slippery mucus that means ovulation is going to take place. This is also the case with the BBT. The BBT won't show a thermal shift unless ovulation happens. When ovulation doesn't take place, there isn't enough progesterone to make the temperature rise. And of course, the cervical opening won't get as wide and feel as soft during times of anovulation as it does around the time of ovulation. In addition, the position of the cervix won't change as much if ovulation doesn't happen.

Basal Body Temperature Patterns During the Anovulatory Cycle

When ovulation does not occur, you will continue to experience a low temperature pattern. This low pattern is just like the one you normally see before ovulation. The thermal shift does not occur. In other words, since ovulation has not taken place, you are unable to apply the Thermal Shift Rule. However, you will be able to use your mucus observations, with special rules discussed later in this chapter, to prevent pregnancy.

The Basic Infertile Patterns of Cervical Mucus

We introduced the Basic Infertile Pattern (BIP) to you in Chapters 5 and 9. Now it's time to look carefully at what this pattern is and what it

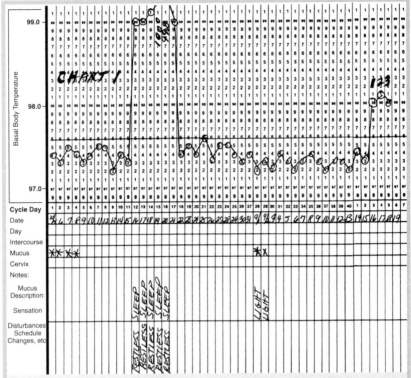

Fig. 44: Delayed ovulation and a delayed thermal shift

LaToya experienced several nights of restless sleep and each morning after these nights, her BBT was in the 99–100°F range. After her sleep returned to normal, her BBT was the usual range that occurs before ovulation. Anne continued to take her BBT, which remained in this low range for almost a month, indicating that she did not ovulate. She experienced some bleeding around the time she usually menstruates, but it was a little lighter and shorter in length than usual. Several days after the bleeding, she experienced a normal thermal shift and applied the Thermal Shift Rule by drawing a line 0.1°F above the highest of the first ten temperatures from her last normal menses. She continued to draw the line all the way across the chart. When the BBT rose above the line for three days, she knew her infertile phase after ovulation had finally begun. You will note this is an interesting situation. LaToya finished completing one chart and had to continue with her fertility sign observations on a second chart. Some women tape their charts together during a time of anovulation so that they can clearly observe the patterns of fertility signs they are recording.

means. The BIP for any woman is the signs she observes while checking her mucus and vaginal sensations that signal to her that she is in an infertile time. The most common BIP for a woman who is ovulating and has fertility cycles that are greater than 25 days in length is the dry day pattern. This means that when menstrual bleeding ends, a woman usually experiences a few to several consecutive dry days. When mucus does appear, this is a signal to the woman that she has probably begun her fertile phase, even if the mucus is the sticky, pasty type. Some women don't have a BIP of dry days. Instead, when menstrual bleeding ends, they experience a few to several consecutive days of non-wet, sticky, pasty mucus and dry and/or sticky vaginal sensations. In this case, the fertile phase begins whenever a woman notices ANY change from her BIP. A change could be an increase in amount, a change in color, and/or a change in the feel of the mucus and vaginal sensations.

As you have learned, a woman can use the Dry Day Rule and have intercourse on the night of any day of her basic infertile pattern, whether this pattern is one of dry days or non-changing mucus days. What do the Dry Day Rule and the BIP have to do with special circumstances? The answer is simple. The Dry Day Rule is a major rule used during special circumstances. When a woman experiences anything in her life that changes her usual time of ovulation, she can safely have intercourse if she is confident in recognizing her BIP. This will become very clear to you as you read about cervical mucus patterns during delayed ovulation and anovulation.

Cervical Mucus Patterns During Delayed Ovulation

When ovulation takes place later than usual in a cycle, the number of days of the BIP usually increases. For example, let's say you menstruate for four days and your usual BIP is dry days after your menstrual bleeding ends. If you usually ovulate between cycle days 12 and 15, you might experience a basic infertile pattern of dry days from cycle day 5 through 9 (Figure 45).

However, if you ovulate later than usual one cycle, let's say around cycle day 20, your basic infertile pattern of dry days will probably last several more days than you are used to experiencing. For example, the dry days could last from cycle day 5 through cycle day 14 (Figure 46)!

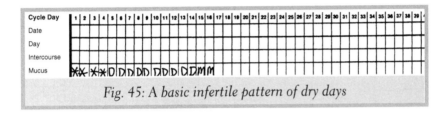

Fig. 45: A basic infertile pattern of dry days

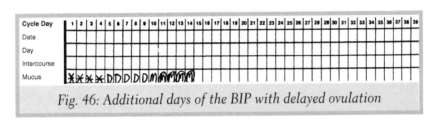

Fig. 46: Additional days of the BIP with delayed ovulation

This means you could have intercourse by applying the Dry Day Rule on all of these days. Your fertile phase would begin as it always has, when there is a change from your BIP. In this case, your BIP is one of dry days, so your fertile phase would begin when you see any type of mucus and/or feel a change in your vaginal sensations. Your fertile phase would end when you could apply the Last Wet Day and Thermal Shift Rules.

Cervical Mucus Patterns During the Anovulatory Cycle

When ovulation does not occur for a while, different qualities of mucus and vaginal sensations can be experienced. The reason for this is that eggs may follow a pattern of growing for a while and then stopping (without ever being released from the ovaries) throughout the entire time of anovulation. When this happens, mucus production is affected in different ways because the amount of estrogen can go up and down during the time a woman does not ovulate. Therefore, if cervical mucus is to be successfully used for the purpose of prevention of pregnancy, it has to be carefully observed and the special circumstances rules followed faithfully.

The different patterns that can be experienced during anovulation are as follows:

❖ You may not produce any mucus and remain dry at the outside of your vaginal area (Figure 47).

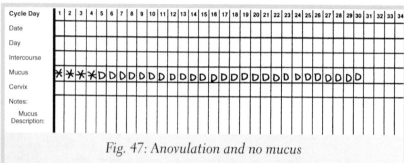

Cycle Day	1	2	3	4	5	6	7	8	9	10	11	12	13	14	15	16	17	18	19	20	21	22	23	24	25	26	27	28	29	30	31	32	33	34
Date																																		
Day																																		
Intercourse																																		
Mucus	✳	✳	✳	✳	✳	D	D	D	D	D	D	D	D	D	D	D	D	D	D	D	D	D	D	D	D	D	D	D	D	D	D			
Cervix																																		
Notes:																																		
Mucus Description:																																		

Fig. 47: Anovulation and no mucus

Jeanine had the flu one cycle, causing a time of anovulation. During the entire time she did not ovulate, she did not see any mucus and a continuous dry vaginal sensation was present.

❖ You may produce non-changing mucus (mucus that remains the same every day for many days). This mucus can be sticky, pasty, and crumbly throughout the entire time you do not ovulate and your vaginal sensations will be dry or sticky. You may produce a wet-feeling mucus with a wet feeling at the outside of your vaginal area throughout the entire time you do not ovulate. The mucus may be of the creamy, wet type or may even feel somewhat slippery and stretchy. However, the mucus will not become the very wet, stretchy, and slippery type that occurs with ovulation. The vaginal sensations will not feel as slippery and lubricated as they usually do with ovulation.

❖ You may experience a combination of changes. For example, you may have dry days and only a few days of sticky, pasty, and crumbly mucus during the entire time you do not ovulate. Or you may experience a mixture of sticky, pasty, and crumbly mucus days; totally dry days; and wet mucus days during the entire time you do not ovulate.

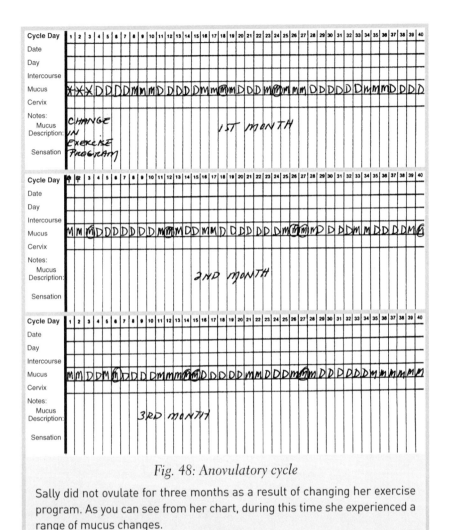

Fig. 48: Anovulatory cycle

Sally did not ovulate for three months as a result of changing her exercise program. As you can see from her chart, during this time she experienced a range of mucus changes.

Cervical Changes During the Anovulatory Cycle

If you have chosen to check your cervix during anovulation, you will find that the cervix can go through various changes. As with mucus, these changes are not predictable and may not follow any specific pattern.

❖ You may experience a low, firm, and closed cervix while you are not ovulating.

* You may experience a slightly raised, slightly soft, and slightly open cervix while you are not ovulating.

* You may even experience a combination of both, low to slightly high, firm to slightly soft, and closed to slightly open.

Bleeding During the Anovulatory Cycle

If you do not ovulate, you may or may not bleed, or spotting of blood may occur. If you do experience bleeding, it may be lighter or heavier than normal, and it may last shorter or longer than your usual menstrual bleeding. The important thing to remember is that *if bleeding of any type occurs during a time of apparent anovulation, it is not necessarily menstrual bleeding. It could be a warning that ovulation is taking place or is going to take place. Therefore, any bleeding is treated as though it is mucus, and a woman should therefore consider herself fertile!*

We have given several possibilities for changes in fertility signs during the anovulatory cycle. Although this may be confusing for some women, when they observe their fertility signs carefully, they can provide themselves with an effective means of family planning.

Anovulation = No Ovulation = A Time of Temporary Infertility

Secondary Signs and Premenstrual Signs During Anovulation

If you usually experience bodily changes that alert you to the approach of ovulation and your menstrual flow, these secondary signs may be different or you may not experience them at all during the time that ovulation does not occur.

Special Circumstances Rules

During times of anovulation, it is very important to remember that **fertility can return at any time**. Since there isn't a way to predict when this will happen, the following special circumstances rules must be followed carefully when you question whether or not you are experiencing either delayed ovulation or anovulation. Since these rules will allow you to see and feel signs of returning fertility, they can be effective in preventing pregnancy.

Dry Day Rule

INTERCOURSE CAN TAKE PLACE ON THE NIGHT OF A DRY DAY.

This is the same Dry Day Rule you have already learned. It states that intercourse may safely occur on the night of any dry day. A dry day means a day of no mucus and a dry vaginal sensation. The day after intercourse may be an abstinence day if a vaginal discharge is observed, because you won't know if it is semen or cervical mucus. Intercourse can continue on the night of each dry day if ovulation is delayed a few days or if a time of anovulation is experienced (Figure 49).

The Mucus Patch Rule

The cervical mucus is the fertility sign that most reliably indicates when a potentially fertile time has started. Therefore, when a woman experiences mucus after having dry days, it may be a signal that her fertility is returning and she is finally going to ovulate again. This is also the case

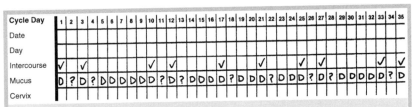

Fig. 49: Use of the Dry Day Rule and anovulation

Diane has not ovulated for two months. Because she has experienced continuous dry days, she has had intercourse by applying the Dry Day Rule. She had to abstain on the days after intercourse because she observed a vaginal discharge on these days (noted with a "?").

if there is a change from a woman's basic infertile pattern of mucus. For example, let's say a woman's basic infertile pattern is sticky, pasty mucus observed for several days in a row. Then one day the mucus changes and feels a bit creamy and slightly wet. The creamy, wet mucus is a change from the woman's BIP. Based on what you know about mucus, we are sure you will agree a change from the BIP could very well be a signal a woman has entered her fertile time and ovulation is going to happen. We are also sure you will agree that the safest choice to make is to abstain when this change begins. The name of the rule to follow when a change from the basic infertile pattern has been experienced is the Mucus Patch Rule.

Mucus Patch Rule

ABSTINENCE FROM INTERCOURSE SHOULD BE FOLLOWED STARTING ON THE DAY ANY TYPE OF MUCUS APPEARS AFTER A BASIC INFERTILE PATTERN OF DRY DAYS HAS BEEN EXPERIENCED.

The appearance of mucus could be an indication that ovulation is going to happen in a few days. Abstinence would be followed during all the days the mucus is observed. If the mucus is a sticky, pasty kind with dry or sticky vaginal sensations, it is highly unlikely ovulation took place because the wet, stretchy, lubricating mucus produced with ovulation was not observed. In this situation, a woman needs to continue to abstain until the mucus is no longer seen and she has returned to her basic infertile pattern of dry days for two consecutive days (see Figure 50 for an exmple of the Mucus Patch Rule). By doing this, she can be sure she did not ovulate, her basic infertile pattern of dry days has resumed, and so the possibility of pregnancy is almost zero.

What if a woman experiences some wet mucus? For example, after she has a few dry days, she observes sticky, pasty mucus that, over the course of a few days, changes into a mucus that is somewhat wet and slippery but never becomes the kind experienced with ovulation. Or let's say the mucus changes to become the classic type of mucus seen with ovulation; however, the woman isn't confident enough in her mucus checking to assume she has ovulated. What should she do? Should she assume ovulation happened and apply the Last Wet Day Rule? This would give her an infertile phase to have intercourse whenever she

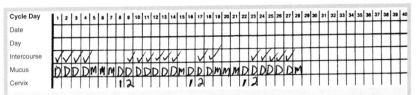

Fig. 50: Using the Mucus Patch Rule with a basic infertile pattern of dry days and non-wet mucus days

In this example, intercourse could occur on the night of any dry day. Abstinence would be followed at the first appearance of non-wet, sticky, pasty mucus that is recorded here with an "M." Abstinence would continue until mucus is no longer seen and two dry days in a row have been experienced. Intercourse could then resume again starting on the night of the second dry day and continue the night of any dry day.

wants. This is probably not the wisest choice. If a woman isn't absolutely confident that she has ovulated (this is where checking BBT is very helpful), she should NEVER assume she has started an infertile phase after ovulation. Therefore, she has to say to herself, "I don't know if I ovulated. I need to continue to observe for mucus and wait until I am confident that ovulation has taken place." In this spirit of careful observation, abstinence needs to be followed until mucus is no longer observed and the basic infertile pattern has been observed for four consecutive days. This is similar to the Last Wet Day Rule in that a woman waits until she has experienced four consecutive days of a basic infertile pattern. The difference is, of course, that the Last Wet Day Rule is used to determine when the infertile phase has begun and ovulation has passed. The Mucus Patch Rule is used to determine when the potentially fertile days have ended because ovulation probably did not take place (Figure 51). Once the rule has been applied, it is safe to resume intercourse on a day-to-day basis while mucus observations are still being made.

As you may have noticed, the Mucus Patch Rule is basically a "wait and see" kind of rule. Abstain when a patch of mucus appears after dry days or when there is a change from a woman's basic infertile mucus pattern. "Wait and see" if the mucus and vaginal sensations give the signal that ovulation has taken place. If not, go back to a "wait and see"

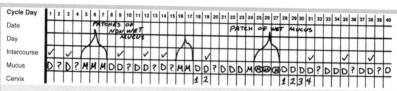

Fig. 51: Using the Mucus Patch Rule during days of non-wet and wet mucus and bleeding

Morgan has not ovulated for over a month and has a basic infertile pattern of dry days, so she has been using the Dry Day Rule for the past 35 days. One day while checking for mucus, she notices the presence of sticky, pasty mucus. Since this could be a sign of approaching ovulation, she begins to abstain. She finds that she has 3 days of the sticky mucus and then returns to experiencing completely dry days. In this situation, Morgan abstains during the 3 days of mucus and for 2 dry days after the mucus ends. Because she did not ovulate, she abstained and waited to see if the following two days were dry. Since they were, she could resume intercourse on the evening of the second dry day.

Morgan continues to use the Dry Day Rule on dry days and the Mucus Patch Rule during pasty, sticky mucus days. One day she notices a wet vaginal sensation and observes wet-feeling mucus. Since ovulation may be near, she abstains during the time when mucus is present. Once the mucus ends, she continues to abstain for 4 dry days instead of 2 dry days. This is because the mucus is wet and that indicates ovulation may have occurred. Because she does not feel confident in assuming that ovulation definitely took place, Morgan follows the Mucus Patch Rule carefully. After applying the Mucus Patch Rule, she can resume using the Dry Day Rule during her completely dry days.

approach. Wait until the basic infertile mucus pattern returns. When it does, abstinence is followed for two consecutive days after the patch of mucus is gone—as long as it never became wet and/or stretchy. If the mucus and/or vaginal sensations did become wet and stretchy, abstinence would need be followed for four days after the BIP resumes. The Dry Day Rule would then be followed carefully (Figure 52 is the chart of a woman who followed these rules).

> *Remember: Always abstain whenever there is a change from the basic infertile pattern of dry days or nonchanging, non-wet mucus or whenever the vaginal sensations change. Again…this*

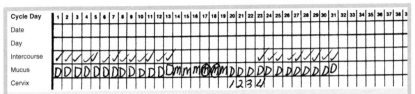

Fig. 52: Using the Mucus Patch Rule conservatively when wet mucus is observed

In this example the first mucus that appears isn't wet, but then it changes into a wet type that becomes stretchy. Abstinence is always followed until the basic infertile pattern of dry days returns. However, because the mucus became wet and ovulation may have taken place, the basic infertile pattern must return for four days. Waiting four days allows time for the life span of one egg, the possibility of a second ovulation, and the life span of the second egg—just as with the Last Wet Day Rule. This is a conservative approach, but we advise following it, just in case ovulation did take place. After four consecutive days of the BIP have been observed, intercourse can then resume on the night of any dry day.

approach is the only one that can be taken during the time a woman is anovulatory. She is always carefully observing her fertility signs so that she will know when her fertility has returned.

Earlier in this chapter, we stated that some women who are not ovulating have a non-changing mucus pattern of wet mucus that can be creamy and perhaps even somewhat stretchy. Figure 53 shows another, though not a particularly common, basic infertile pattern. As you might imagine, this can be a tricky BIP to use to prevent pregnancy. A woman with this type of BIP has to carefully look for any change in the already wet mucus and vaginal sensations to a wetter mucus or one that has a different color, stretchiness, and a feeling of wetness. When she notices this, she must abstain and follow the Mucus Patch Rule. She would wait until her BIP returns for four consecutive days before resuming intercourse on the night of any day of her BIP. Actually, there is no research that has followed a significant number of women with this type of BIP to determine the effectiveness of the Mucus Patch and Dry Day Rules.

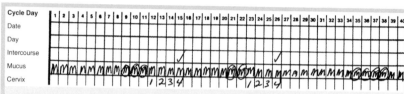

Fig. 53: Using the Mucus Patch Rule conservatively with a basic infertile pattern of non-changing mucus

In this example, the basic infertile pattern is non-changing, non-wet, pasty, sticky mucus. Intercourse can occur on the night of any nonchanging mucus day. At the moment there is a change from the BIP to any type of wet-feeling mucus, abstinence would be followed. Abstinence would then continue until the change in unusual mucus is no longer observed and the BIP of non-changing mucus has been experienced for four consecutive days. When this happens, intercourse can then be resumed on the night of BIP day.

The key is that the woman herself must feel completely confident in using this type of BIP with the special circumstances rules to prevent pregnancy.

TO REVIEW

1. When using the **Mucus Patch Rule** with a basic infertile pattern of **dry days**, you must abstain on any day that you experience any type of mucus and/or wet, slippery vaginal sensations. The mucus or sensations could mean that ovulation is approaching.

   If the mucus you experience after a dry day is sticky, pasty, and crumbly, and vaginal sensations are dry, you need to abstain during the days when mucus is present and for two dry days after the mucus goes away. Then you can resume applying the Dry Day Rule.

   If the mucus feels wet and vaginal sensations are wet and slippery, you need to abstain during those days when the mucus is present and until four consecutive dry days after the wet mucus goes away. Then you can resume applying the Dry Day Rule. For an example of how these rules should be used when a woman has a BIP of dry days, see Figure 52.

2. When using the Mucus Patch Rule with a basic infertile pattern of non-changing non-wet mucus days (Figure 54), you must abstain if you experience any change from the BIP. Continue to abstain until the change

in mucus is gone and the basic infertile pattern of nonchanging non-wet mucus has been experienced for four consecutive days. Then you can resume applying the Dry Day Rule.

Bleeding and Anovulation

If any type of bleeding occurs during a time of anovulation, these days are treated as though they are potentially fertile days. This is for the same reasons that the most conservative NFP rules recommend abstaining from intercourse during menstrual bleeding. Bleeding makes it difficult if not impossible to observe mucus accurately. In addition,

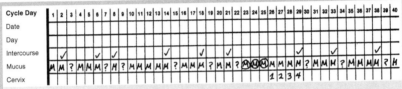

Fig. 54: Using the Dry Day Rule and Mucus Patch Rule with a basic infertile mucus pattern

Marlene has been experiencing anovulation for three months. During this time she has observed a basic infertile pattern of sticky, pasty, and non-wet mucus day after day, so she has been using the Dry Day Rule on these days. One day she notices the mucus has changed. It now feels wet. This could be a sign of the approach of ovulation. Because of this she abstains during the days of the wet mucus. However, the mucus never became the very slippery, stretchy mucus with slippery, lubricating vaginal sensations that is experienced with ovulation. Therefore, Marlene assumes she did not ovulate. As soon as the mucus has returned to its basic infertile pattern of the non-wet, sticky, and pasty type for four days in a row, she can resume using the Dry Day Rule.

there have been instances in which a woman who hasn't ovulated for a while bleeds, and during bleeding she is actually ovulating! Because of this and the difficulty in seeing mucus when blood is present, it makes sense to abstain during any days of bleeding. The question is, what if ovulation occurred during bleeding? What if it even happened on the last day of bleeding? Is it safe to resume intercourse the day after

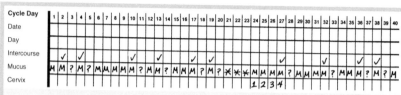

Fig. 55: *Anovulation, the Mucus Patch Rule, and bleeding*

Rosa has not been ovulating for 3 months. During this time, she has been having intercourse on the evening of her BIP. During the fourth month of anovulation, Rosa experiences bleeding. Since this could mean ovulation is occurring, she abstains during the bleeding. As soon as the mucus has returned to its basic infertile pattern for four days after the bleeding ends, she can resume using the Dry Day Rule.

bleeding ends? Probably not. To be most conservative, because the egg could still be in the fallopian tube waiting for sperm on the day after bleeding, it is best to continue to abstain until the basic infertile pattern has been experienced for four days after the bleeding ends (Figure 55). If ovulation cannot be proven to have happened during the bleeding, it is best to resume intercourse on the night of any dry day or basic infertile mucus pattern.

In reality, since it is difficult if not impossible to check mucus during bleeding, what is the best way to prove ovulation has taken place? It is, of course, observing a thermal shift occurring during bleeding or shortly after the bleeding has ended. Once again, this is the value of taking the BBT. It is a wonderful fertility sign to use in combination with mucus checking to help a woman confirm that she has ovulated. The question some women ask about the BBT is, "Does it need to be taken every day during a time of anovulation?" The answer is no. If taking the BBT every day during anovulation is a problem for some women, those women can choose to take the BBT only when they notice a change from their basic infertile pattern or any bleeding. This way they can use the BBT to confirm ovulation without having to take it every day. If a woman experienced such a change, she would take her BBT every day during the change and for four days after the change. If she didn't see a

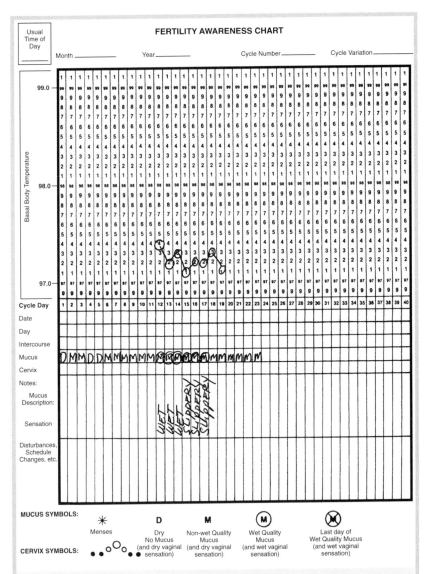

Fig. 56: Using the BBT with the BIP to see if ovulation has occurred

In this example, the BBT was taken when the mucus changed from its BIP of non-wet, sticky, pasty mucus to become wet mucus and, later, slippery and stretchy mucus. As you will notice, the BBT did not rise. It remained low, indicating ovulation probably did not occur.

clear thermal shift, she knows that she probably did not ovulate (see the example in Figure 56). She can then stop taking her BBT until she again experiences a change from her BIP.

What to Do When Normal Fertility Returns

Once ovulation returns, you can, of course, use any of the NFP rules you choose except for the 21 Day Rule. This rule should not be used until ovulation has definitely returned for six cycles in a row.

Why Can There Be Bleeding During Anovulation?

It may seem strange that a woman could bleed but not ovulate, and that she could even bleed around the time she experienced menstrual bleeding with past cycles. The probable explanation for this is that an egg begins to grow for a while, and because of this, estrogen is being produced. As estrogen increases, it causes more blood to flow into the lining of the uterus. When the egg stops growing, the lining no longer continues to thicken with blood. Eventually the blood that was stored in the lining flows out of the vagina. This is anovulatory bleeding. Anovulatory bleeding is usually lighter and/or lasts fewer days than the normal menstrual bleeding. This is because the lining doesn't usually become filled with as much blood as it does when an egg completely matures and is released from the ovary.

Why Can There Be Bleeding with Ovulation?

The reason for spotting or bleeding with ovulation is not as well understood. Around the time of ovulation, progesterone, when combined with the estrogen being made, should keep the entire lining in place. For some reason, this doesn't happen for some women, and a very small area of the lining doesn't stay in place. This allows some blood to leave. It is important to know that if the bleeding isn't heavy, this doesn't usually mean there is a problem or that a woman will have difficulty become pregnant in the future. However, if it happens more than two cycles in a row, it would be a good idea to discuss this with a clinician.

Causes of Anovulation

Although anovulation may last indefinitely, ovulation will usually return. When it does, you will observe the thermal shift and the very wet, slippery, stretchy mucus with the slippery, lubricated vaginal sensations. The Thermal Shift Rule and Last Wet Day Rule can then be applied to determine the beginning of the infertile phase after ovulation.

Anovulation has many causes. An illness with a fever is just one; some other causes include:

HEALTH PROBLEMS, MEDICAL TREATMENTS, AND MEDICATIONS

There is no way that anyone can predict the effects of many health problems, medications, or treatments on the time of ovulation or a woman's fertility pattern. It depends on the problem, how it affects the woman's body, and her emotional state. Therefore, the most helpful and honest statement we can make about this problem is that if one should arise, no matter how minor (even a cold!), always carefully observe your fertility signs to see how your body adapts to the problem. If you experience a specific health issue that requires you be under the care of a health-care professional, please discuss the possible effects it might have on your fertility. This is true of any medication you may be advised to take. Sometimes even undergoing a surgical procedure that has nothing to do with the reproductive system (such as having the tonsils removed) could affect ovulation, because it is still a shock to the body.

There are other health issues that affect a woman's fertility for more obvious reasons. Once such example is a thyroid imbalance, since this major gland helps keep everything in the body in balance. Sometimes having a health problem that causes pain—let's say an injured back— can cause anovulation. Why? Because the woman's body and mind is trying to deal with constant pain. This could cause changes in hormones in the brain and chemicals in different parts of the body. The changes could end up affecting the ovaries and stop ovulation for a while. Being emotionally upset by being in pain can have similar effects. As you can imagine, we could discuss any number of ways in which various health issues can affect fertility. However, there are several books available that are devoted to discussing fertility, should you be interested in learning more about this topic. We have included the names of a few of these in the Bibliography.

HORMONAL METHODS OF CONTRACEPTION

Any hormonal method of contraception that contains estrogen and/or progestin works to prevent pregnancy primarily by stopping ovulation. This includes birth control pills, the contraceptive patch, monthly injections, and the contraceptive ring. Once you stop using these methods of contraception, ovulation may begin within two to three weeks or may not begin for months. There are other hormonal methods that contain only progestin. These include the progestin-only birth control pill, the progestin-only injection, and the progestin-treated intrauterine system. After a woman stops using a progestin-only contraceptive method, ovulation can begin within a few weeks or may be delayed for up to a few months. Usually, a woman's ovulation pattern returns to the pattern it followed before she began the method. This means that if she did not ovulate regularly before using the method, there is a good chance she will return to not ovulating regularly after she stops the method. The good news is that a woman's fertility is rarely affected in any negative way by any hormonal method.

Sometimes, however, even when ovulation begins soon after the hormonal method is no longer being used and a thermal shift is observed, the cervical mucus doesn't reveal the usual pattern that indicates ovulation is taking place. It may take a month or more for the cervix to respond to the hormone changes and therefore to return to making a normal ovulatory mucus pattern. In other words, some women see a thermal shift, but the mucus does not seem to become the very wet, slippery, stretchy mucus. Should this happen, the Last Wet Day Rule cannot be used. Instead, the Thermal Shift Rule can be used alone with a minimal possibility of pregnancy.

CHANGE IN DIET AND/OR EXERCISE ROUTINE

Any change in life can affect a woman's fertility. When a woman changes her eating habits and/or exercise routine, for reasons not always understood, ovulation may be delayed for a week or so or even stop for a while. Sometimes a 5–10-pound weight gain or loss can cause a change in the ovulatory pattern or can cause anovulation. A change in diet and/or exercise without a weight loss or gain can also have the same effect. Once the body becomes adjusted to this change in weight, exercise, or nutrition, ovulation usually returns.

PERIMENOPAUSE

As a woman approaches her late 30s to her mid-40s, she will usually experience gradual changes in her fertility cycle. She may not ovulate every month. For example, she may ovulate every two to three months or even less frequently. She may also experience a change in the amount of menstrual bleeding and the number of days it lasts. Her period may be longer or shorter and the bleeding may be lighter or heavier. All of these changes signal that the ovaries are starting to make less estrogen and progesterone. This indicates that a woman is approaching the end of her fertile years and is called the perimenopause (before menopause). The perimenopause lasts for a few to several years. After menstrual bleeding has stopped for twelve consecutive months, the possibility of ovulating is rare. In fact, once this has happened, a woman is said to have reached her menopause. This is the time in which there are very few immature eggs left in her ovaries. These eggs are no longer able to grow because of the aging process. At this point, she can no longer become pregnant.

Since a woman approaching menopause may ovulate infrequently and have times of delayed ovulation, she should use the special circumstances rules, just as any other woman who is experiencing delayed ovulation or anovulation. She would use the Dry Day and Mucus Patch Rules during the times of anovulation. When she does ovulate, she can apply the Thermal Shift and Last Wet Day Rules to determine the infertile phase after ovulation. A woman ovulating infrequently should not use the 21 Day Rule. She can use the menses rule only if she is sure she ovulated during the previous cycle. If this is the case, she can also use the dry day rule until she begins to observe mucus. She would then apply the rules most appropriate to her situation.

EMOTIONAL STRESS

The way you feel emotionally can affect your body physically. Over the past few years the relationship between the mind and the body has been studied a great deal. It is well known that emotional stress can cause ulcers, backaches, and headaches. All of us experience stressful events in our lives: changing jobs, a death in the family, travel, family visits, and on and on. Any of these may cause you to not ovulate for a month or more.

DEVELOPMENT OF AN OVARIAN CYST

Occasionally, the developing egg may not continue to the point of ovulation. Instead, the capsule it grows in enlarges to form a cyst on the ovary, lasting about two to six weeks. Usually ovulation does not occur while the cyst is present. Another type of cyst can develop in the ovary after ovulation, and it also lasts about two to six weeks. During the time the cyst is present, irregular bleeding may be experienced or the menstrual period can be delayed a week or more. Some women experience pain as well. These are common cysts that usually go away on their own. However, there are other, less common, cysts that don't go away on their own, so it is important that any woman who misses her period, experiences pain, or has irregular bleeding be examined. Irregular bleeding and pain can also be caused by a pregnancy, either in the uterus or inside or outside one of the fallopian tubes.

In the case of a common ovarian cyst that causes a change in the time of ovulation, as with all other causes of delayed ovulation and anovulation, the Dry Day Rule and Mucus Patch Rule are used until ovulation returns.

BREASTFEEDING

During breastfeeding, ovulation may occur irregularly or not at all. This usually depends upon the way a woman chooses to breastfeed.

Some women breastfeed their babies at least every four hours during the daytime and at least every six hours at night. If they begin this schedule of breastfeeding soon after the baby is born and have not started any type of bleeding, this breastfeeding schedule causes what is called lactational amenorrhea. This is the name for having no menstruation (amenorrhea) because of breastfeeding (lactation). Research has shown that with lactational amenorrhea, a woman's chance of becoming pregnant for up to six months after the baby is born is only about 1 percent. In fact, when this type of breastfeeding pattern is followed for pregnancy prevention it is called the Lactational Amenorrhea Method (LAM) for pregnancy prevention. The method works so well because the chances of a woman ovulating are very small. To use LAM effectively,

- Breastfeeding must occur at least once every four hours during the daytime.
- Breastfeeding must occur at least every six hours at the night.
- The woman must not have begun menstruating.
- The baby must be six months of age or younger.
- No supplements should be given to the baby (except perhaps a minimal amount of liquid).

If a woman breastfeeds her baby in any other way, no one can predict when she will or will not ovulate. Giving the baby water, juice, or other types of nourishment, or even allowing the baby to suck on a pacifier, can increase a woman's chance of ovulating as compared to her chances if she follows LAM strictly. If any changes occur during breastfeeding that lead to the baby feeding at the breast less often or for shorter amounts of time, a woman must remember that this can cause ovulation to return within a short period of time.

The decision of how and why to breastfeed will depend upon many factors, including whether you are working or involved in other activities that prevent you from being with the baby throughout the day. Unfortunately, some women have been told that if they breastfeed once or twice a day, they will not ovulate and cannot become pregnant. This is not true for most women. The return of ovulation is affected by the amount of suckling that occurs throughout the day. The less often the baby has an opportunity to suckle at the breast each day, the greater the chance of ovulation.

The return of ovulation, and therefore fertility, will vary from woman to woman. In general, the earliest return of ovulation for a woman who is breastfeeding exclusively (using LAM) is about 10 weeks after delivery. The *average* return of ovulation for a woman who is breastfeeding exclusively (using LAM) is about 14½ months after delivery. When a woman bottle-feeds her baby, pumps her breasts, or breastfeeds without meeting the LAM criteria, ovulation can begin within 2–4 weeks after delivery. Unless a woman is following LAM carefully, it is not unusual for a woman to become pregnant within a month or two of delivering her baby! Therefore, we recommend breastfeeding mothers observe their mucus carefully.

In general, a woman who is breastfeeding may experience one or more of these mucus patterns:

1. She may only have dry days during the entire time of exclusive breastfeeding.

2. She may experience one or more days of crumbly, pasty, sticky mucus between dry days.

3. Occasionally a woman who is breastfeeding exclusively may also experience wet sensations and wet mucus, usually of the more creamy type. This type of mucus can be present between dry days or days of crumbly, pasty, sticky mucus. The possibility of this happening is unlikely, unless she is experiencing a change in her breastfeeding pattern.

4. If there is any change in the breastfeeding pattern—be it caused by the introduction of supplemental liquids or baby food, a baby who cannot or will not breastfeed as long or as often, or a mother who, because of work or other reasons, cannot breastfeed the baby as often or as long—*fertility can return at any time.* When this happens, a woman will notice changes in her mucus pattern. When the changes begin and what the pattern will actually look and feel like can't be predicted. For example, a woman might begin to breastfeed her baby less and within two weeks notice the appearance of sticky,

pasty mucus. Perhaps up to that point she has had a BIP of dry days only. She may continue with this type of mucus and dry vaginal sensations for a long time. However, she may not, and instead right away experience wet mucus that becomes slippery. She may or may not ovulate when this happens. She could experience any number of mucus changes until she finally ovulates. As the baby breastfeeds less and less, the body will try harder and harder to ovulate until it succeeds. During this process the woman can experience several "patches of mucus"—days of different kinds of mucus between dry days.

5. Days of bleeding may even occur. Since mucus could be mixed in with the blood, *it is very important to treat the days of bleeding—even slight spotting—as fertile mucus days and to abstain from intercourse.*

The breastfeeding woman who is either not ovulating or ovulating occasionally needs to follow the Dry Day and Mucus Patch Rules. If you are interested in learning more about using breastfeeding as a method of birth control, we suggest reading *Natural Breastfeeding and Child Spacing* by Sheila Kippley. (See the Natural Family Planning section of the Bibliography for information about this book.)

Vaginal Dryness During Anovulation

Some women who breastfeed and some women who are approaching menopause experience dryness of the vaginal tissues. The loss of the usual moisture in these tissues is due to a lack of the estrogen that is usually present in large amounts when a woman is ovulating. If the vaginal tissues become dry, intercourse and urination can be uncomfortable or painful. A woman should talk with her health-care provider if this happens. Sometimes a vaginal estrogen cream is helpful, as is a vaginal moisturizer such as Replens, or any of the great vaginal lubricants that are available in drugs stores and grocery stores. If a lubricant doesn't help, estrogen cream is often used to prevent tearing and infection of the tissues. The breastfeeding woman may be advised to decrease the number of times she is breastfeeding the baby in order to stimulate eggs to grow. This will cause more estrogen to help heal the vaginal tissues. Of course, this will mean the return of fertility sooner than she may have wanted, not to mention weaning the baby earlier than she had planned.

Will dry vaginal tissue affect mucus traveling down to the vaginal opening? It may, since moist vaginal tissue can help the mucus travel at a faster rate than dry tissue allows it to travel. Again, this is an area in which research is sorely lacking. Because some NFP experts believe this may be the case, it is of course very important that all mucus rules used during times of anovulation be carefully followed. Moist vaginal tissue probably helps cervical mucus travel down to the vaginal opening. Dry vaginal tissue probably does not aid the flow of mucus.

A reminder about basal body temperature for new mothers, women approaching menopause, and all other women experiencing anovulation: We realize that taking the basal body temperature every day may not be convenient. If the temperature cannot be taken every day, as previously mentioned, we strongly suggest taking it as soon as there is an appearance of wet mucus or a change from the basic infertile pattern. If the thermal shift occurs when there has been a mucus pattern that changes to ovulatory, wet, stretchy, lubricating mucus and vaginal sensations, the Thermal Shift and Last Wet Day Rules can be applied to determine the beginning of the infertile phase after ovulation. However, until a woman has resumed ovulating for six cycles in a row, the 21 Day Rule cannot be applied.

For example, Carmen has ovulated for the first time after one year of breastfeeding. She is now able to use the Thermal Shift and Last Wet Day Rules. Yet until her fertility signs give proof of ovulation for six cycles, she should consider herself fertile during any type of bleeding, unless she is sure she ovulated during the previous cycle. In this case she could use the Menses Rule during the first five days of her fertility cycle. When bleeding ends, she should follow the Dry Day Rule. When any mucus appears, she should begin to abstain until she has applied the Last Wet Day and Thermal Shift Rules to determine the beginning of the infertile phase after ovulation.

You will be able to recognize anovulation and prevent pregnancy through careful observation of fertility signs. Missing periods for a few months in no way harms the body. However, if you do not ovulate for more than one month and you are not breastfeeding, we suggest you discuss this situation with your doctor. Occasionally, anovulation can be a sign of a medical problem, such as improper functioning of the thyroid gland. It is therefore important to attempt to determine the cause of anovulation. The good news is that most of the time, anovulation occurs because the woman's body is responding to changes in lifestyle. Ovulation usually returns when the body gets used to the changes.

TO REVIEW

BASAL BODY TEMPERATURE

- A woman who ovulates will see her temperature shift from low to high.
- A woman who does not ovulate will not see her temperature shift from low to high.

CERVICAL MUCUS

- A woman who ovulates will develop very wet, slippery, stretchy, lubricating mucus and very lubricated, slippery vaginal sensations as she approaches ovulation.
- A woman who does not ovulate can experience a variety of mucus patterns, from all dry days to a combination of different mucus changes. However, her mucus will not have the same quality as mucus that is seen with ovulation.

CERVICAL CHANGES

- A woman who ovulates will experience a cervix that rises to a high position, becomes soft, and opens wide.
- A woman who does not ovulate will experience a cervix that either remains low, firm, and closed or that rises slightly and becomes slightly soft and slightly open.

SECONDARY FERTILITY SIGNS

- A woman who is not ovulating will probably not experience her usual secondary fertility signs.

Remember, if you have anovulatory cycles that continue beyond one month, it is important to discuss this with your health-care provider. It is also helpful to take your fertility awareness charts to this person, since reviewing the charts can help him or her to better understand your particular situation.

Other Special Circumstances

After Childbirth

If you are not breastfeeding, you may begin ovulating within two weeks after the delivery. If you want to use your fertility signs to prevent pregnancy, you should begin observing your mucus and temperature as soon after the delivery as possible. It can be difficult for you to observe your fertility signs if you are a new mother, since you are awakening at irregular times to take care of your new baby, and so on. However, you should try to begin checking your mucus when the lochia, the discharge from childbirth, has stopped. Usually, by three weeks after delivery the lochia will no longer be present and observation of the mucus can begin. By that time you should also try to begin taking your temperature.

Vaginal Infection

Another common special circumstance affecting the use of NFP is a vaginal infection. One of the symptoms of a vaginal infection is the presence of a discharge that looks different from normal vaginal secretions and cervical mucus. The second symptom can be an odor in the vaginal area that is unlike the usual vaginal scent. A third symptom can be burning and/or itching in the vaginal area. If you experience any symptoms of a vaginal infection, it is important for you to be examined to identify the cause of the infection and receive proper treatment.

During the time of a vaginal infection you will probably have difficulty observing your mucus because of the abnormal discharge and the presence of vaginal medication, if you are using one. However, you can still continue to take your basal body temperature. It is not advisable to check your cervix (if that is your usual practice), nor to have intercourse, until the vaginal infection has cleared up. This allows the delicate vaginal tissues to heal well from the infection. If intercourse continues during an infection, symptoms can be made worse. Vaginal tissue can become seriously infected and it will take longer for the area to heal completely. If the infection is healed by the time you have accurately applied the Thermal Shift Rule, you can safely resume intercourse.

Premenstrual Syndrome

As previously discussed, premenstrual syndrome (PMS) is the name given to various troubling emotional and/or physical changes associated with the menstrual period. The symptoms can last anywhere from 1–14 days, sometimes beginning shortly after ovulation, but more often being experienced a few days before the period begins. (Some women also seem to experience the changes only during menstruation and for a couple of days after menstruation ends.)

There are over one hundred different symptoms associated with PMS. The most common symptoms are nervous tension, mood swings, irritability, anxiety, headache, craving for sweets, increased appetite, heart pounding, fatigue, dizziness, forgetfulness, crying, confusion, insomnia, weight gain, swelling of hands, feet, and legs, breast tenderness, and abdominal bloating.

Research in the field of PMS is limited, but it has shown that PMS is clearly caused by several factors and has a real physical basis. There doesn't seem to be one cause of PMS, nor one cure-all treatment. PMS symptoms may be due to imbalances in various hormones, including estrogen and progesterone, that cause changes in brain chemistry and the way other glands function. An imbalance in hormones affects every part of the body to some degree, including brain chemistry—that is the reason for many of the emotional changes experienced with PMS.

We have included the names of a few books on PMS in the Bibliography, because PMS is a real problem that rarely goes away on its own. It can negatively affect the quality of a woman's life and can worsen as the years go by. What is important to know is that there is much a woman can do to help treat the symptoms and perhaps even the causes of PMS.

We have included some treatment recommendations below and encourage you, if you have PMS, to consider learning more about it and embarking on a health program that will help you feel better.

Does PMS Affect the Use of NFP and FAM?

Picture the woman who has applied the Last Wet Day and Thermal Shift Rules and has begun her infertile phase after ovulation. She resumes having intercourse or puts her method of birth control away, only to find that within a few days after ovulation she begins to experience breast tenderness, bloating, headaches, and fatigue. Does she now feel like having intercourse? Perhaps not! In other words, the woman following NFP or FAM who experiences PMS may have an infertile phase after ovulation partially or totally filled with physical and/or emotional changes that cause her to not want to engage in any kind of sexual activity. What then does the infertile phase after ovulation have to offer her if she is unable to use it to enjoy her sexual life?

In addition to affecting how a woman feels, PMS may affect her fertility signs. We have observed slow rising temperature patterns, irregular mucus patterns, and temperatures that do not remain elevated during the usual 12–16 day time period from ovulation to menstrual bleeding. No one knows whether PMS causes slight or severe irregularities in the fertility sign patterns of every woman who has it. However, what *is* known is that a woman can help herself feel better, and if her fertility signs are affected, they will probably be easier to identify if her PMS is being treated successfully.

Some Final Tips on Special Circumstances and Mucus

Some women have stated that when they have decreased the amount of mucus-producing foods (for example, dairy foods) in their diets, they have noticed a decrease in the amount of cervical mucus produced.

Other women who have needed to take prescription antihistamines, drugs that dry up the secretions in the nasal passages, notice a drying up of their mucus.

You can become aware of the factors that might affect your own mucus pattern. If you change your diet or need to take certain drugs and see a change from your mucus pattern, with careful observation you will probably still be able to observe your mucus signs to avoid pregnancy. If you experience a substantial decrease in mucus or a constant dry feeling, yet you know you are ovulating by seeing a thermal shift, you might have to rely on all the rules that don't require mucus checking. These are the Twenty One Day, Menses, and Thermal Shift Rules. If this continues for over two cycles, it is important to consider talking with your health-care provider about this situation. It may also be valuable to seek advice from a fertility awareness instructor.

✤ ✤ ✤

As you can see from the different life situations we have discussed, just about every woman can observe her fertility signs as a means of pregnancy prevention. If you experience a special circumstance, be on the lookout for mucus changes as the primary sign of the beginning of a potentially fertile time and the return of ovulation. Follow the special circumstances rules carefully. Please remember that the language of fertility your body speaks is a clear, accurate language. The time and effort you spend will enable you to understand it. We hope you will be encouraged, for the language is worth the learning.

11

The Fertility Awareness Method

Barrier and spermicidal methods are effective family planning options used by many couples. Barrier methods include male and female condoms, the diaphragm and the cervical cap, and are effective because they prevent sperm from traveling up into the cervix. Spermicides are substances that destroy sperm before they have a chance to travel into the cervix. These include vaginal film, cream, jelly, foam, and suppositories. Another barrier method, the sponge, will probably be available again one of these days.

The traditional way of using barrier and/or spermicidal methods is to use them every time intercourse takes place. However, when you think about it, they only need to be used when a woman can become pregnant—during her fertile time!

Couples who have been using barrier and spermicidal methods finally have an alternative. They don't have to use these methods every time they have intercourse. Instead, they can use the fertility awareness method (FAM). This method is based on the same scientific principles as natural family planning, but FAM is for those who do not wish to abstain from intercourse during the fertile days of the fertility cycle and would like to decrease the number of days barrier or spermicidal contraceptive methods have to be used.

A couple having intercourse during the fertile phase can use any of the barrier or spermicidal methods mentioned above, and then put them away during the infertile days.

The way in which FAM is used depends upon the contraceptive method(s) you choose to use and the fertility sign(s) you are comfortable observing. For example, Judy has been using the diaphragm for two years. Although she is basically satisfied with it, she and her partner have been talking about changing their method of birth control to one that does not interrupt their lovemaking. They feel that at times the diaphragm does not allow them the freedom they would like to have with intercourse. This couple decided to give FAM a chance, and Judy learned how to determine her fertile and infertile phases. Once she learned this, she and her partner no longer needed to use the diaphragm each time they had intercourse. Now that they need to use the diaphragm less often, they no longer feel the need to change their method of birth control.

HOW CAN YOU MINIMIZE THE USE OF BIRTH CONTROL METHODS AFTER OVULATION? We have already discussed the factors that can prevent you from accurately observing your cervical mucus. One of these factors is spermicides. When spermicide is in the vagina, it mixes with the cervical mucus and makes accurate observation of mucus impossible. Therefore, if you choose to use a spermicide, you will be unable to observe your mucus changes during the days when the spermicide is present in your vagina. However, the fertility sign that *can* be observed is your basal body temperature.

The basal body temperature can be used with or without cervical changes. Observation of the basal body temperature and use of the Thermal Shift Rule can provide you with a great way to identify the infertile phase after ovulation. Once this phase begins, the barrier and/or spermicidal method does not have to be used until the infertile phase ends and the next cycle begins.

For example, a woman can use a diaphragm or cervical cap (a spermicide must be used with these methods), a female condom (a lubricant must be used with it), or a spermicide alone from the first day of her cycle until she can apply the Thermal Shift Rule. Once the infertile phase begins, she no longer needs to use the method for the remainder of that fertility cycle. Knowing when the infertile phase after ovulation begins eliminates the need for birth control for about ten days of the fertility cycle.

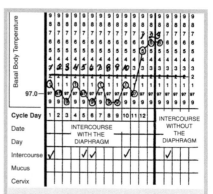

Another example of how FAM can be applied is the use of the nonlubricated condom in combination with cervical mucus and basal body temperature observations. Because the condom prevents semen from entering the vagina, the cervical mucus is not affected. Use of the condom allows accurate observation of mucus changes and successful application of all the mucus rules. The Menses and Dry Day Rules can be followed, and condoms would not need to be used

Fig. 57: Diaphragm use and the Thermal Shift Rule

Laura used her diaphragm whenever she had intercourse until she applied the Thermal Shift Rule. Beginning on the evening of the third high temperature above the coverline and throughout the remainder of that cycle, Laura could have intercourse safely without needing her diaphragm.

on days that are safe according to these rules. When mucus observations indicate the fertile phase has begun, the condom would be used if intercourse were to take place. When the Last Wet Day and Thermal Shift Rules are applied, the condom would not have to be used for the remainder of the cycle.

HOW CAN YOU MINIMIZE THE USE OF BIRTH CONTROL METHODS BEFORE OVULATION? The 21 Day and Menses Rules can be used just as they are used with NFP. The Dry Day Rule can also be followed if nonlubricated condoms are the method of choice.

Here are some typical cases:

If your last six fertility cycles were 30, 31, 30, 29, 30, and 29 days long, by subtracting 21 from the shortest of the six cycles you determine that you have an infertile phase before ovulation of 8 days $(29 - 21 = 8)$.

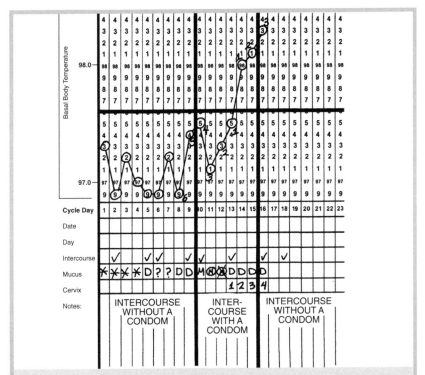

Fig. 58: Condom use and the 21 Day and Thermal Shift Rules

Chris was able to apply the 21 Day Rule, which gave her an infertile phase of 9 days before her fertile phase starts. During that time she and Nick had intercourse without using a method of contraception. Since they wished to have intercourse after the start of the fertile phase on day 10, they used nonlubricated condoms. Use of these condoms enabled them to observe the cervical mucus changes. They continued to use a condom until they could apply the Last Wet Day and Thermal Shift Rules. Once the infertile phase began on the evening of cycle day 16, they continued having intercourse, but without having to use condoms for the remainder of that fertility cycle.

On the first 8 days of your fertility cycle you can feel free to have intercourse without another method of birth control. When the fertile phase begins, if you choose to have intercourse, you can use a spermicide and/or barrier method until you can successfully apply the Thermal Shift Rule (and, if possible, apply the Last Wet Day Rule). Once the infertile phase after ovulation begins, you no longer need to use your other method of birth control for the remainder of the fertility cycle.

To reduce the risk of pregnancy during the infertile phase before ovulation and the fertile phase, the Menses Rule and the Dry Day Rule can be used, as explained in Chapter 9. The Dry Day Rule can only be applied if you are able to check for the presence or absence of mucus. The nonlubricated condom is the only contraception method that enables you to watch for the presence of early warning mucus, which could indicate an earlier- or later-than-usual ovulation.

As you can see, fertility signs, NFP rules, and other methods of birth control can be combined in a variety of ways to avoid pregnancy.

Contraceptive methods can be used during the fertile phase only. They can also be used before the fertile phase begins and during the infertile phase after ovulation. As with NFP, the rule(s) used will depend on how great the desire is to prevent pregnancy, weighed against the desire to decrease the number of times a barrier and/or spermicidal method needs to be used.

As discussed in Chapter 2, it is generally believed that the pregnancy rates with FAM should not be any higher than the pregnancy rates for using the barrier and/or spermicidal methods alone, provided the rules are followed carefully.

Your willingness to observe your fertility signs and use the birth control methods conscientiously are the key to FAM. Because intercourse is taking place during the fertile phase—the phase with the highest risk of pregnancy—the careful and consistent use of the contraceptive methods is of utmost importance if pregnancy is to be prevented. It is extremely important to consider using a spermicide during the fertile phase if male condoms are your method of choice for the infertile times. Condoms can break and fall off. Having a spermicide in the vagina is an added measure of protection should it be needed. A couple using a diaphragm or cervical cap might want to consider adding the condom if they are going to have intercourse during the fertile phase. Again, this serves as added protection in the event that the diaphragm or cervical cap moves out of place.

If a condom does break or the other barrier methods move out of place, even when a spermicide is used, it is important to remember that emergency contraceptive pills (ECPs) are available through many pharmacists, physicians, and local family planning, department of health, or Planned Parenthood clinics. These are not the abortion pill, but a hormone pill very much like the birth control pill that can reduce the chances of pregnancy if an emergency situation arises, such as a condom breaking. They must be taken within seventy-two hours from the time of the emergency situation (having intercourse with a method failure). If a woman is already pregnant, they will not harm the pregnancy. For more information about ECPs, you can call (888) NOT-2LATE.

YOUR NOTES

12

The Advantages and Disadvantages of Natural Family Planning and Fertility Awareness Methods

The majority of this book has been about facts—facts about the reproductive organs, the fertility cycle, and fertility signs and rules. We hope what you have learned has been valuable for you and that you will be able to use all of these facts in many rewarding ways.

Having correct information about your fertility can help you discover how you *feel* about yourself, your sexuality, and pregnancy. That is what this chapter is about: feelings—feelings about fertility and sexuality—and what these feelings mean to you. This is of great importance, because your feelings will determine what the possible advantages and disadvantages of natural family planning or the fertility awareness method will be for you.

Should You Use Natural Family Planning?

A conscious decision to use NFP, or any method of family planning for that matter, is one that only you can make. Taking time to examine the advantages and disadvantages that NFP has for you personally will help you to answer the very important question of whether or not you should use it as your method of family planning.

Advantages...

❖ NFP is not physically harmful.

❖ It promotes an understanding of the fertility cycle.

❖ It can be used by the woman who has irregular fertility cycles, is breastfeeding, or is perimenopausal.

❖ It is as effective in preventing pregnancy, if used properly, as most other birth control methods.

❖ The man joins in a mutual sharing of responsibility for fertility control.

❖ NFP can promote a greater understanding of one another's sexual and emotional needs. This can enhance a couple's love and respect for each other.

❖ Alternative forms of sexual pleasuring can be experienced during the fertile days.

❖ In addition, it is an inexpensive means of family planning.

Disadvantages...

❖ NFP initially requires more time to learn and use than other family planning methods.

❖ It requires the cooperation of the man.

❖ It may require a change in sexual lifestyle, since abstinence during the fertile days is necessary.

❖ NFP offers no protection from sexually transmitted diseases.

Please keep in mind that what may be experienced as an advantage for some may be a disadvantage for others. For example, if the man finds it difficult to abstain during the fertile days and is not supportive of fertility sign observation and charting, then the relationship may be disrupted. If the man wants to use NFP and the woman finds it difficult to abstain during the fertile days, the relationship may also be disrupted.

However, when there is mutual commitment to abstinence, the relationship is often enhanced.

If you are considering NFP as a method of pregnancy prevention, an important question to ask yourself is: Can I reach a mutual agreement with my partner to abstain from intercourse periodically and feel good about this way of preventing pregnancy?

For some, this may be a difficult question. It can be helpful to consider whether in your relationship you are able to talk together openly and honestly about how to prevent pregnancy. If your relationship is one in which effective and satisfying communication about sexuality and birth control cannot occur, it does not mean it will always be that way. In a relationship a man and woman learn, grow, and change. And fortunately, there are ways to help the growing process so people can experience and enjoy the kinds of relationships they want.

With so many social changes taking place so rapidly in our society, there is a great opportunity for women and men to learn about themselves and their sexuality. This new awareness can enable them to make more responsible decisions than ever before.

What Does Sexuality Mean?

For some, sexuality only means intercourse—an activity for the main purpose of babymaking. For others, it means a variety of ways of physical pleasuring. And for still others, it has a different meaning, including more than sexual activity. This broader definition includes all of the physical and emotional aspects of being a man or a woman, such as the way a person walks, talks, dresses, and makes love, and even the type of work someone does.

Keeping this broader definition in mind, let's take a look at how we learn about sexuality. Learning about sexuality begins at birth and continues throughout our lifetime. This learning is influenced by everything and everyone around us. Unfortunately, much of the learning involves information that is usually incorrect or incomplete. We often receive messages that our genitals are "dirty" and that sex is something to be hidden. As children, perhaps we tried to learn what sex was all about. Often this learning was done in secret—behind the garage, in the attic, or in the basement. Then, as puberty approached, our bodies began to change. These changes, such as menstruation, breast development, sexual feelings, wet dreams, pubic hair, and acne, often created uncomfortable and even frightening feelings.

Somehow, as if by magic, in adolescence we were expected to have healthy, mature attitudes about our bodies, our sexuality, and ourselves. Finally, as adults we are expected to be knowledgeable, sensitive, and comfortable about sexuality, and to take responsibility for our sexuality and fertility. This is not easy when so many of us received a great deal of misinformation and many negative messages about our sexuality.

Misinformation and negative messages are major reasons why people either do not use birth control, or use it improperly. For example, a woman and man who are uncomfortable about their own sexuality often do not take responsibility for preventing pregnancy, even though they are having intercourse. When an accidental pregnancy occurs, many women say, "I didn't know it (intercourse) was going to happen," or "I didn't think I could get pregnant." The man often says, "It was her fault. She should have done something to prevent the pregnancy."

Misinformation and negative messages not only contribute to unplanned pregnancies, they can also lead to sexual concerns and difficulties. These concerns include many types of dissatisfaction during lovemaking, from the woman who wants an orgasm but doesn't achieve one, to the man who is unable to have or keep an erection.

Other common reasons for sexual dissatisfaction are disagreements about the times to make love, how long lovemaking should last, and the type of sexual activity that occurs. For example, a woman may prefer sex in the morning, while her partner may prefer sex in the evening.

It is estimated that nine out of ten couples experience dissatisfaction at some time during their relationship because of a lack of accurate information about sex and the failure of the woman and man to discuss their feelings and, if necessary, seek professional guidance.

When uncertain of the facts about sex, people are often afraid to discuss it. Asking questions about sex and talking with a partner, doctor, friend, or counselor can be difficult. A person may fear sounding foolish or abnormal in some way. To some, talking with a partner means acknowledging unhappiness with their lovemaking. Because of this, a person may be afraid that his or her partner will feel hurt or become angry.

What we are saying is that there are very real reasons why people aren't open with their feelings about sexuality. But this doesn't mean they shouldn't try to open up. Once women and men begin to talk about their feelings, they are often amazed to find that their partners have many of the same questions and fears. By sharing these thoughts they become closer, and this helps to enhance not only their sexual lives but other aspects of their relationship as well.

Many couples have also found that by talking, planning, and agreeing on how they want their sexual life to be, they set aside time for giving each other attention and pleasure.

Do You Want a Pregnancy?

This is one of the major questions related to fertility and sexuality that doesn't get asked or decided on as frequently as it should be. The answer to this question is determined by many factors, since people decide to have children for different reasons.

There are many reasons why people want children. Some of the reasons can be disruptive to the relationship, while others lead to the development of a loving and happy family.

* "To share our love with another human being"
* "We have so much to give"
* "A woman isn't a woman until she has a child"
* "A man isn't a man until he has a child"
* "To have someone to love"
* "To carry on the family name"

❖ "To give our parents grandchildren"

❖ "It's normal and expected"

Some men and women see a child as a solution to a problem in their lives.

❖ "Having a baby will keep us together"

❖ "Having a baby will keep my wife in her place"

❖ "Having a baby will make my husband happy, even if I don't want a child right now"

❖ "Nothing seems to help these lonely feelings I have"

❖ "I'm nothing unless I am a mother/father"

Having a child can be one of the most wonderful and gratifying experiences in life. Yet the decision to have a child should not be taken lightly. It requires a great deal of thought, for it is about whether or not a couple have reached a time in their lives when they are able to care for and truly love each other, as well another human being.

Just as there are many reasons why people choose to have a child, there are also many reasons why couples choose to avoid having a child, at least for a period of time.

❖ "I can't emotionally provide for another person at this time in my life"

❖ "I feel emotionally fulfilled with the child/children I have"

❖ "Having a child right now would take time away from developing our relationship"

❖ "I need to go to school."

❖ "I want time to develop my career."

❖ "I can't afford to have a child."

The decision to prevent a pregnancy or to become pregnant may be difficult to make. Yet it must be made consciously if any method of birth control is to be used effectively.

When a couple have not firmly decided upon a birth control method, there are certain situations in which unplanned pregnancies commonly occur. These include a holiday, vacation, a romantic evening, and an occasion where drugs or alcohol are used. When people are relaxed and not feeling the stress in their lives, life's responsibilities and demands do not seem as great, and the desire for sexual pleasure can be increased. In these situations women often become pregnant. Unfortunately, after the vacation is over or the effects of the alcohol have worn off, the stresses of real life return, and the pregnancy is often viewed as a tragedy.

Unplanned pregnancies occur frequently not only during the situations described above, but also at times when a woman or man is experiencing major life changes. Such changes include a separation from a marriage or relationship, graduation from high school or college, dissatisfaction with a job or career, feelings of loneliness, or other times of unhappiness. All too often, men and women think that having a child will be the answer to these problems.

We've discussed some facts about sexuality, reasons people have for preventing and achieving pregnancy, as well as a few of the situations in life that commonly lead to unplanned pregnancy.

Sexuality and fertility play a major role in determining who we are and what we do. And as with all good things, sometimes there are problems. The reassuring point is that working out the problems can be a rewarding and positive experience.

How Does Natural Family Planning Fit into All of This?

Many couples who make the choice to abstain from intercourse during their fertile days say that sharing in this method has been an enriching experience for their relationship. Many women not involved in a sexual relationship with one particular person find that using fertility signs to avoid pregnancy gives them a sense of control over their bodies and reproduction. They also find that when their partner learns more about how they avoid pregnancy, he is often fascinated by it, desires to learn more, and is supportive of the method.

By discussing their feelings, some men and women find that abstinence from intercourse—and even all sexual activity—during their fertile time works perfectly for them. Others discover that they choose to enjoy their partners sexually in ways other than intercourse.

Expressing sexuality without having intercourse brings up other issues about the use of NFP. Abstinence, in its true definition, means not having intercourse. For some it also means not experiencing other forms of sexual pleasuring, such as oral sex and other forms of sensual touching. For others it means that fertile days can be sexually enjoyable times without experiencing intercourse. It becomes a time for touching, massaging, caressing, and enjoying any type of physical contact that a man and woman feel comfortable with. Others who find sexual contact—without intercourse—during fertile times difficult, frustrating, or against their beliefs, find that they are able to share love, affection, and enjoyable times without sexual activity.

In fact, it is sad to say—but great to know—that couples often experience a rebirth in their relationship when they can't have intercourse whenever they desire to. By "sad to say," we mean that it is not unusual for a couple to fall into a routine in which they forget to compliment each other, do things for one another, and, in general, enjoy each other without sex. Women and men have commented that becoming aware of fertility and sharing the responsibility of birth control in their sexual relationship has given them a new view of their relationship and their reasons for being together—a new awakening, so to speak. For many, this new and greater understanding has enhanced their love for each other.

The Advantages of the Fertility Awareness Method

The use of FAM involves all that we have discussed above, plus a bit more. Many couples feel that abstinence seems unnatural to them and isn't compatible with their lives. Others feel that if a fertile time coincides with a vacation, holiday, birthday, or just a day when the woman or man feels sexual, they want to be able to have intercourse, yet do not want a pregnancy to result. Many are comfortable with the use of the diaphragm, cervical cap, male or female condom, or spermicide and also feel that they benefit from not feeling tied down to these methods each time they have intercourse. FAM offers a choice for them.

A Few Last Words...

We hope that you have enjoyed *Natural Birth Control Made Simple* and through it have learned exciting, interesting, and helpful information. After reading about fertility, some people find that they wish to have the information reinforced for them, or want the opportunity to share particular questions and concerns with someone knowledgeable about the information. If you find this is true for you, there are various ways to locate such a person. One way is through a fertility awareness or natural family planning class. Though there may not be such classes in all areas of the country, by contacting a church group, your state department of public health, or a family planning or local Planned Parenthood organization, you can learn what instructors and/or physicians are available to help you.

It is impossible in one short book about fertility awareness to provide all of the available information about sexuality, communication, and relationships. However, we wanted to give you some food for thought and encouragement so that, if you haven't already, you will begin to do what is important for you—to feel that you deserve to make your own decisions as to how you will meet your family planning needs and enjoy your sexual life in ways that are best for you. We are discovering more and more that, regardless of age, type of relationship, or how men and women choose to use fertility awareness information, it has enabled them to learn about themselves and each other.

Through this learning process, many couples are sharing feelings and mutual responsibility for enjoying their sexuality. They have learned to feel comfortable about the role fertility plays in their lives. We hope you will, too.

Sample NFP Contracts

The thought of a birth control contract may sound cold and impersonal or perhaps even strange to you. Or it may be an exciting concept.

We have chosen to include it because some women and men have found that it helps them to talk with one another in order to make decisions concerning their sexual lives and feelings about pregnancy and birth control.

The nice part of the contract is that it is negotiable. This means that the couple can change it at any time! Let's say one of the partners in a relationship is feeling as though she/he wants to have a child, when six months ago the person felt quite the opposite. The contract can be pulled out and discussed, and perhaps changed. In fact, the contract probably should be discussed every six months or so, since this can be a helpful way to regularly assess one's personal needs and family planning goals.

On the next two pages are examples of two such contracts for use in natural family planning. If they don't quite suit your needs, feel free to adapt them or to write one of your own.

Sample Contract for the Woman

I understand that if this method is to work, I must use it carefully and correctly.

Because I know there are many reasons for taking chances and allowing pregnancy to happen, I will always explore, try to understand, and, if I choose, communicate my feelings about what a pregnancy means to me.

I understand that to prevent a pregnancy means

+ no intercourse during the fertile days
+ no other sexual activity that causes semen to come into contact with my vaginal area during the fertile days

Because I respect myself and am aware of my responsibility to myself, I agree to abide by this contract.

Should problems arise with the use of the method, or should I change my mind about avoiding pregnancy, I will decide how to best meet my needs and change the contract accordingly.

by:

_____   _____
SIGNATURE   DATE

Please note, for women who are concerned about being exposed to a sexually transmitted disease, it is important that they take precautions to prevent this from happening. The most conservative approach is to avoid all genital-to-genital contact unless a female or male condom is being used.

Sample Contract for the Couple

We understand that if this method is to work, we must use it carefully and correctly.

Because we know that there are many reasons for taking chances and allowing a pregnancy to happen, we will always explore, try to understand, and communicate our feelings about what a pregnancy means to us.

We understand that to avoid a pregnancy means

+ no intercourse during the fertile time
+ no other sexual activity that causes semen to come into contact with the vaginal area during the fertile days

Should problems arise with the use of the method, or should one of us change his/her mind about avoiding pregnancy, we will discuss this with each other and mutually agree upon how the contract should be changed.

by:

_____   _____
SIGNATURE   DATE

by:

_____   _____
SIGNATURE   DATE

Please note, for people who are concerned about being exposed to a sexually transmitted disease, it is important that they take precautions to prevent this from happening. The most conservative approach is to avoid all genital-to-genital contact unless a female or male condom is being used.

Bibliography

NATURAL FAMILY PLANNING

Billings, John J., M.D. *The Ovulation Method: Natural Family Planning.* Collegeville, MN: Liturgical Press, 1992.

Kippley, Sheila K. *Breastfeeding and Natural Child Spacing: How Ecological Breastfeeding Spaces Babies.* Cincinnati, OH: Couple to Couple League Intl., 1999.

FERTILITY AND INFERTILITY

Berger, Gary S., M.D., et al. *The Couple's Guide to Fertility.* New York: Broadway Books, 2001.

Marrs, Richard P., M.D. *Dr. Richard Marrs' Fertility Book.* New York: Delacorte Press, 1997.

Silber, Sherman J., M.D. *How to Get Pregnant with the New Technology.* New York: Warner Books, 1998.

WOMEN'S HEALTH

Boston Women's Health Book Collective. *Our Bodies, Ourselves for the New Century: A Book by and for Women.* New York: Simon & Schuster, 1998.

Goldberg, Burton. *Alternative Medicine Guide to Women's Health.* New York: Alternative Medicine, 2000.

Hankinson, Susan E., Sc.D., et al.(eds.) *Healthy Women, Healthy Lives: A Guide to Preventing Disease from the Landmark Nurses' Health Study.* New York: Simon & Schuster, 2001.

Smith, Kathy. *Kathy Smith's Moving Through Menopause: The Complete Program for Exercise, Nutrition, and Total Wellness.* New York: Warner Books, 2002.

PREMENSTRUAL SYNDROME

Bender, Stephanie Degraff. *PMS: Women Tell Other Women How To Control Premenstrual Syndrome.* Oakland, CA: New Harbinger, 1996.

Dalton, Katharina, M.D. *Once a Month: Understanding and Treating PMS.* Alameda, CA: Hunter House, 1999.

Harrison, Michelle, M.D. *Self Help for Premenstrual Syndrome.* New York: Random House, 1999.

Moe, Barbara. *Coping with PMS.* New York: Rosen Publishing, 2002.

Murray, Michael T. *Premenstrual Syndrome: How You Can Benefit from Diet, Vitamins, Minerals, Herbs, Exercise, and Other Natural Methods.* Rocklin, CA: Prima Publishing, 1997.

EXERCISE

Bach, Marilyn L., Ph.D., and Schleck, Lorie, M.A., P.T. *ShapeWalking: Six Easy Steps to Your Best Body.* Alameda, CA: Hunter House, 2003.

Callahan, Lisa, M.D. *Fitness Factor: Every Woman's Key to a Fitness Lifetime of Health and Well-being.* Guilford, CT: Lyons Press, 2002.

Nelson, Miriam E., Ph.D. *Strong Women Stay Young.* New York: Bantam Books, 2000.

Parker, Margaret Hundley. *KISS Guide to Fitness.* New York: DK Publishing, 2002.

Yap, Chan Ling, Ph.D. *Fusion Fitness: Combining the Best from East and West.* Alameda, CA: Hunter House, 2003.

NUTRITION

Brand-Miller, Jennie, Ph.D., et al. *The Glucose Revolution Life Plan.* New York: Marlowe & Co., 2001.

Kesten, Deborah. *The Healing Secrets of Food: A Practical Guide for Nourishing Mind, Body, and Soul.* Novato, CA: New World Library, 2001.

Heber, David, M.D. *What Color is Your Diet? The 7 Colors of Health.* New York: Regan Books, 2001.

Nelson, Miriam E., Ph.D. *Strong Women Eat Well: Nutritional Strategies for a Healthy Body and Mind.* New York: Putnam's, 2001.

STRESS REDUCTION

Adamson, Eve. *The Everything Stress Management Book: Practical Ways to Relax, Be Healthy, and Maintain Your Sanity.* Avon, MA: Adams Media Corp, 2002.

Seaward, Brian Luke. *Stressed Is Desserts Spelled Backward*. York Beach, ME: Conari Press, 1999.

Sieg, Diane, R.N. *Stop Living Life Like an Emergency: Rescue Strategies for the Overworked and Overwhelmed*. New York: Lifeline Press, 2002.

Singh Khalsa, Dharma, M.D. *Meditation as Medicine: Activate the Power of Your Natural Healing Force*. New York: Pocket Books, 2001.

Witkin, Georgia, Ph.D. *Stress Relief for Disasters Great and Small: What to Do from Day One to Year One and Beyond*. New York: Newmarket Press, 2002.

SEXUALITY

Craze, Richard. *The Pocket Book of Foreplay*. Alameda, CA: Hunter House, 1999.

———. *The Pocket Book of Sensational Orgasms*. Alameda, CA: Hunter House, 2003.

Hooper, Anne. *KISS Guide to Sex*. New York: Dorling Kindersley, 2000.

———. *Anne Hooper's Sexual Intimacy: How to Build a Lasting and Loving Relationship*. New York: Dorling Kindersley, 1996.

Hutcherson, Hilda, M.D. *What Your Mother Never Told You About S.E.X.* New York: Putnam's, 2002.

Keesling, Barbara, Ph.D. *Rx Sex: Making Love Is the Best Medicine*. Alameda, CA: Hunter House, 2000.

———. *Sexual Pleasure: Reaching New Heights of Sexual Arousal and Intimacy*. Alameda, CA: Hunter House, 1993.

Laken, Virginia, and Laken, Keith. *Making Love Again: Hope for Couples Facing Loss of Sexual Intimacy*. East Sandwich, MA: Ant Hill Press, 2002.

McCarthy, Barry, and McCarthy, Emily. *Sexual Awareness: Couple Sexuality for the 21st Century*. New York: Carroll & Graf, 2002.

Stein, Daniel S., M.D. *Passionate Sex: Discover the Special Power in You*. New York: Carroll & Graf, 2000.

Swift, Rachel. *How to Have an Orgasm...As Often As You Want*. New York: Carroll & Graf, 2001.

Williamson, Marvel L., Ph.D., RN. *Great Sex After 40: Strategies for Lifelong Fulfillment*. New York: Wiley, 2000.

Index

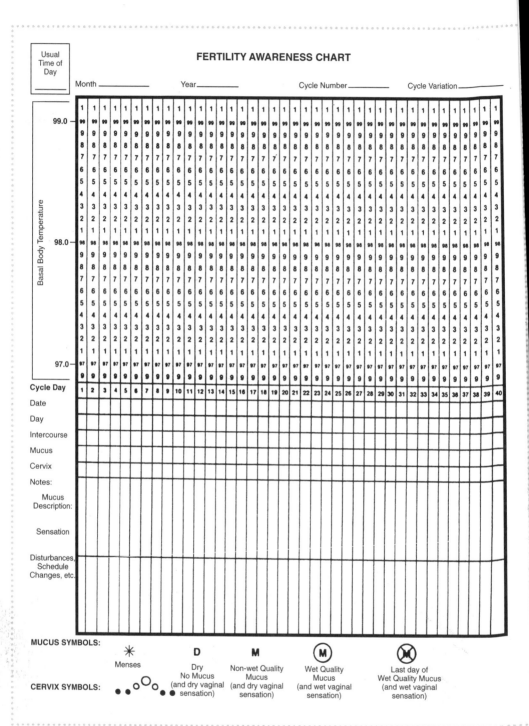

FERTILITY AWARENESS CHART

Usual Time of Day _____

Month _____ Year_____ Cycle Number_____ Cycle Variation_____

MUCUS SYMBOLS:

✳	D	M	Ⓜ	Ⓧ
Menses	Dry No Mucus (and dry vaginal sensation)	Non-wet Quality Mucus (and dry vaginal sensation)	Wet Quality Mucus (and wet vaginal sensation)	Last day of Wet Quality Mucus (and wet vaginal sensation)

CERVIX SYMBOLS: ● ● ○ ○ ○ ●

From *Natural Birth Control Made Simple* by Barbara Kass-Annese, RN, MSN and Hal C. Danzer, MD. ©2003. This chart maybe reproduced for personal use—fits on lettersize paper when enlarged 150%. Also may be downloaded in pdf format from www.hunterhouse.com. To reorder call 1-800-266-5592.